Biomarkers of Neuroinflammation

PROCEEDINGS OF A WORKSHOP

Lisa Bain, Noam I. Keren, and Sheena M. Posey Norris,
Rapporteurs

Forum on Neuroscience and
Nervous System Disorders

Board on Health Sciences Policy

Health and Medicine Division

The National Academies of
SCIENCES · ENGINEERING · MEDICINE

THE NATIONAL ACADEMIES PRESS
Washington, DC
www.nap.edu

THE NATIONAL ACADEMIES PRESS 500 Fifth Street, NW Washington, DC 20001

This activity was supported by contracts between the National Academy of Sciences and the Alzheimer's Association; Brain Canada Foundation; Cohen Veterans Bioscience; the Department of Health and Human Services' Food and Drug Administration (5R13FD005362-02) and National Institutes of Health (NIH) (HHSN26300089 [Under Master Base #DHHS-10002880]) through the National Center for Complementary and Integrative Health, National Eye Institute, National Institute of Mental Health, National Institute of Neurological Disorders and Stroke, National Institute on Aging, National Institute on Alcohol Abuse and Alcoholism, National Institute on Drug Abuse, and NIH Blueprint for Neuroscience Research; Department of Veterans Affairs (VA240-14-C-0057); Eli Lilly and Company; Foundation for the National Institutes of Health; The Gatsby Charitable Foundation; George and Anne Ryan Institute for Neuroscience at The University of Rhode Island; Janssen Research & Development, LLC; Lundbeck Research USA; Merck Research Laboratories; The Michael J. Fox Foundation for Parkinson's Research; National Multiple Sclerosis Society; National Science Foundation (BCS-1064270); One Mind; Pfizer Inc.; Pharmaceutical Product Development, LLC; Sanofi; Society for Neuroscience; and Takeda Development Center Americas, Inc. Any opinions, findings, conclusions, or recommendations expressed in this publication do not necessarily reflect the views of any organization or agency that provided support for this project.

International Standard Book Number-13: 978-0-309-46365-2
International Standard Book Number-10: 0-309-46365-3
Digital Object Identifier: https://doi.org/10.17226/24854

Additional copies of this publication are available for sale from the National Academies Press, 500 Fifth Street, NW, Keck 360, Washington, DC 20001; (800) 624-6242 or (202) 334-3313; http://www.nap.edu.

Copyright 2018 by the National Academy of Sciences. All rights reserved.

Printed in the United States of America

Cover image courtesy of Dr. Gary Landreth, Case Western Reserve University, Cleveland, Ohio.

Suggested citation: National Academies of Sciences, Engineering, and Medicine. 2018. *Biomarkers of neuroinflammation: Proceedings of a workshop*. Washington, DC: The National Academies Press. doi: https://doi.org/10.17226/24854.

The National Academies of
SCIENCES · ENGINEERING · MEDICINE

The **National Academy of Sciences** was established in 1863 by an Act of Congress, signed by President Lincoln, as a private, nongovernmental institution to advise the nation on issues related to science and technology. Members are elected by their peers for outstanding contributions to research. Dr. Marcia McNutt is president.

The **National Academy of Engineering** was established in 1964 under the charter of the National Academy of Sciences to bring the practices of engineering to advising the nation. Members are elected by their peers for extraordinary contributions to engineering. Dr. C. D. Mote, Jr., is president.

The **National Academy of Medicine** (formerly the Institute of Medicine) was established in 1970 under the charter of the National Academy of Sciences to advise the nation on medical and health issues. Members are elected by their peers for distinguished contributions to medicine and health. Dr. Victor J. Dzau is president.

The three Academies work together as the **National Academies of Sciences, Engineering, and Medicine** to provide independent, objective analysis and advice to the nation and conduct other activities to solve complex problems and inform public policy decisions. The National Academies also encourage education and research, recognize outstanding contributions to knowledge, and increase public understanding in matters of science, engineering, and medicine.

Learn more about the National Academies of Sciences, Engineering, and Medicine at **www.nationalacademies.org**.

The National Academies of
SCIENCES · ENGINEERING · MEDICINE

Consensus Study Reports published by the National Academies of Sciences, Engineering, and Medicine document the evidence-based consensus on the study's statement of task by an authoring committee of experts. Reports typically include findings, conclusions, and recommendations based on information gathered by the committee and the committee's deliberations. Each report has been subjected to a rigorous and independent peer-review process and it represents the position of the National Academies on the statement of task.

Proceedings published by the National Academies of Sciences, Engineering, and Medicine chronicle the presentations and discussions at a workshop, symposium, or other event convened by the National Academies. The statements and opinions contained in proceedings are those of the participants and are not endorsed by other participants, the planning committee, or the National Academies.

For information about other products and activities of the National Academies, please visit www.nationalacademies.org/about/whatwedo.

PLANNING COMMITTEE ON BIOMARKERS OF NEUROINFLAMMATION[1]

RITA BALICE-GORDON (*Co-Chair*), Sanofi
LINDA BRADY (*Co-Chair*), National Institute of Mental Health
BRIAN CAMPBELL, MindImmune Therapeutics, Inc.
ROSA CANET-AVILES, Foundation for the National Institutes of Health
TIMOTHY COETZEE, National Multiple Sclerosis Society
RICHARD HODES, National Institute on Aging
STUART HOFFMAN, Department of Veterans Affairs
ELIEZER MASLIAH, National Institute on Aging
PATRICIO O'DONNELL, Pfizer Inc. (*until March 2017*)
WILLIAM POTTER, National Institute of Mental Health
RICHARD RANSOHOFF, Biogen
BETH STEVENS, Harvard Medical School
STEVIN ZORN, MindImmune Therapeutics, Inc.

Health and Medicine Division Staff

CLARE STROUD, Forum Director
SHEENA M. POSEY NORRIS, Program Officer
NOAM I. KEREN, Associate Program Officer
DANIEL FLYNN, Senior Program Assistant
ANDREW M. POPE, Director, Board on Health Sciences Policy

---

[1] The National Academies of Sciences, Engineering, and Medicine's planning committees are solely responsible for organizing the workshop, identifying topics, and choosing speakers. The responsibility for the published Proceedings of a Workshop rests with the workshop rapporteurs and the institution.

FORUM ON NEUROSCIENCE AND NERVOUS SYSTEM DISORDERS[1]

STEVEN HYMAN (*Chair*), Broad Institute of Massachusetts Institute of Technology and Harvard University
STORY LANDIS (*Vice Chair*), Director Emeritus, National Institute of Neurological Disorders and Stroke
SUSAN AMARA, Society for Neuroscience
RITA BALICE-GORDON, Sanofi
KATJA BROSE, Chan Zuckerberg Initiative
EMERY BROWN, Harvard Medical School and Massachusetts Institute of Technology
DANIEL BURCH, Pharmaceutical Product Development, LLC
JOSEPH BUXBAUM, Icahn School of Medicine at Mount Sinai
SARAH CADDICK, The Gatsby Charitable Foundation
ROSA CANET-AVILES, Foundation for the National Institutes of Health
MARIA CARRILLO, Alzheimer's Association
E. ANTONIO CHIOCCA, Harvard Medical School
TIMOTHY COETZEE, National Multiple Sclerosis Society
JONATHAN COHEN, Princeton University
FAY LOMAX COOK, National Science Foundation
BILLY DUNN, Food and Drug Administration
JOSHUA GORDON, National Institute of Mental Health
HANK GREELY, Stanford University
RAQUEL GUR, University of Pennsylvania
MAGALI HAAS, Cohen Veterans Bioscience
RAMONA HICKS, One Mind
RICHARD HODES, National Institute on Aging
STUART HOFFMAN, Department of Veterans Affairs
MICHAEL IRIZARRY, Eli Lilly and Company
INEZ JABALPURWALA, Brain Canada Foundation
FRANCES JENSEN, University of Pennsylvania
GEORGE KOOB, National Institute on Alcohol Abuse and Alcoholism

---

[1] The National Academies of Sciences, Engineering, and Medicine's forums and roundtables do not issue, review, or approve individual documents. The responsibility for the published Proceedings of a Workshop rests with the workshop rapporteurs and the institution.

WALTER KOROSHETZ, National Institute of Neurological Disorders and Stroke
ALAN LESHNER, American Association for the Advancement of Science (Emeritus)
HUSSEINI MANJI, Janssen Research & Development, LLC
DAVID MICHELSON, Merck Research Laboratories
JAMES OLDS, National Science Foundation
ATUL PANDE, Tal Medical
STEVEN PAUL, Voyager Therapeutics, Inc.
RODERIC PETTIGREW, National Institute of Biomedical Imaging and Bioengineering
EMILIANGELO RATTI, Takeda Pharmaceuticals International
TAREK SAMAD, Pfizer Inc.
TODD SHERER, The Michael J. Fox Foundation for Parkinson's Research
DAVID SHURTLEFF, National Center for Complementary and Integrative Health
PAUL SIEVING, National Eye Institute
NORA VOLKOW, National Institute on Drug Abuse
DOUG WILLIAMSON, Lundbeck
STEVIN ZORN, MindImmune Therapeutics, Inc.

Health and Medicine Division Staff

CLARE STROUD, Forum Director
SHEENA M. POSEY NORRIS, Program Officer
NOAM I. KEREN, Associate Program Officer
DANIEL FLYNN, Senior Program Assistant
JIM BANIHASHEMI, Financial Officer
HILARY BRAGG, Program Coordinator (*until August 2017*)
ANDREW M. POPE, Director, Board on Health Sciences Policy

Reviewers

This Proceedings of a Workshop was reviewed in draft form by individuals chosen for their diverse perspectives and technical expertise. The purpose of this independent review is to provide candid and critical comments that will assist the National Academies of Sciences, Engineering, and Medicine in making each published proceedings as sound as possible and to ensure that it meets the institutional standards for quality, objectivity, evidence, and responsiveness to the charge. The review comments and draft manuscript remain confidential to protect the integrity of the process.

We thank the following individuals for their review of this proceedings:

KATERNIA AKASSOGLOU, University of California,
  San Francisco
ELIEZER MASLIAH, National Institute on Aging
THOMAS MÖLLER, AbbVie Foundational Neuroscience Center
TAREK SAMAD, Pfizer R&D

Although the reviewers listed above provided many constructive comments and suggestions, they were not asked to endorse the content of the proceedings nor did they see the final draft before its release. The review of this proceedings was overseen by **JOSEPH T. COYLE,** Harvard Medical School. He was responsible for making certain that an independent examination of this proceedings was carried out in accordance with standards of the National Academies and that all review comments were carefully considered. Responsibility for the final content rests entirely with the rapporteurs and the National Academies.

Contents

1 Introduction and Overview   1
Workshop Objectives, 3
Organization of the Proceedings, 3

2 Biomarkers of Neuroinflammation: Challenges and Potential Opportunities   5
Overview of Challenges, 5
Overview of Potential Opportunities, 8

3 State of the Science of Neuroinflammation in Central Nervous System Disorders   15
Microglia and Neuroinflammation, 16
Synaptic Pruning, 19
Blood–Brain Barrier Dysfunction, 20
Fibrinogen and the Neurovascular Interface, 22

4 Neuroinflammation in Disease   25
Multiple Sclerosis, 26
Traumatic Brain Injury, 28
Huntington's Disease, 30
Alzheimer's Disease, 31
Immunopsychiatry, 33

5 Neuroimaging Biomarkers: Current Initiatives and Opportunities   37
Nuclear Imaging Approaches, 39
Magnetic Resonance Imaging Approaches, 40

6 Cerebrospinal Fluid and Other Fluid Biomarkers: Current Initiatives and Opportunities   45
Novel Approaches to Identifying Genetic and Molecular Markers of Neuroinflammation, 48

7 Potential Mechanisms for Moving Forward   51
Consortial Efforts to Identify and Validate Biomarkers of Neuroinflammation, 54

APPENDIXES

A	References	57
B	Workshop Agenda	63
C	Registered Attendees	71

1

Introduction and Overview[1]

Neuroinflammation is a burgeoning area of interest in academia and biopharma with a broadly acknowledged role in many central nervous system (CNS) disorders, said Rita Balice-Gordon, head of neuroscience research at Sanofi, Inc. However, she added, there is little agreement on the pathophysiological mechanisms that underlie the manifestations of neuroinflammation in the CNS compartment and how neuroinflammation operates as a driver and also as a consequence of disease in the brain. Moreover, another unclear area is how to translate increased understanding of the mechanisms that underlie neuroinflammation and its manifestations in the CNS to therapeutics. In particular, she cited the need for biomarkers that can be used as markers, not only of disease progression but of therapeutic efficacy as well, to make clinical trials and regulatory paths more straightforward.

To address these gaps in understanding mechanisms and how to translate that understanding into therapeutics, the Forum on Neuroscience and Nervous System Disorders of the National Academies of Sciences, Engineering, and Medicine convened a workshop on March 20-21, 2017, bringing together key leaders in the field from industry, academia, and governmental agencies to explore the role and mechanisms of neuroinflammation in a variety of CNS diseases. The workshop also considered strategies to advance the identification and validation of biomarkers of neuroinflammation that could accelerate development of therapies, bringing much-needed treatments to patients with disorders ranging from neuroinflammatory diseases, such as multiple sclerosis (MS), to neuropsychiatric disorders, such as depression (see Box 1-1).

---

[1] The planning committee's role was limited to planning the workshop, and the Proceedings of a Workshop was prepared by the workshop rapporteurs as a factual summary of what occurred at the workshop. Statements, recommendations, and opinions expressed are those of individual presenters and participants, and are not endorsed or verified by the National Academies of Sciences, Engineering, and Medicine, and they should not be construed as reflecting any group consensus.

BOX 1-1
Statement of Task

An ad hoc committee will plan and conduct a 1.5-day public workshop that will bring together key stakeholders from government, academia, industry, and disease-focused organizations to explore and advance efforts to identify biomarkers of neuroinflammation that can be validated and used in clinical development and regulatory decision making.

Invited presentations and discussions will be designed to:

- Provide an overview of current knowledge on the role of neuroinflammation in nervous system disorders—including psychiatric and neurological disorders, neurodevelopmental disorders, and neurodegeneration resulting from traumatic brain injury.
- Discuss the various definitions of neuroinflammation in use across the field, and the contribution of the peripheral and central nervous system's innate immune systems to normal brain function and disease pathophysiology.
- Explore the state of the science of neuroinflammation biomarkers and research needed to enable the use of these biomarkers at the individual level. Do any biomarkers under development/validation implicate glia, neurons, immune cells, or endothelial cells? Should these be deployed singly or in combination, and where are the gaps in current approaches?
- Facilitate coordination among consortia and companies that are developing biomarkers of neuroinflammation. How might a study be designed to establish the disease relevance or drug development utility of a neuroinflammation biomarker? Are such studies under way, and if not, why not? If not, what more do we need to facilitate these, and are there opportunities for "add-on" studies to current clinical trials?
- Highlight approaches, tools, and lessons learned that may apply across disorders and opportunities to advance the development of these biomarkers.

The committee will develop the agenda for the workshop, select and invite speakers and discussants, and moderate the discussions. A summary of the presentations and discussions at the workshop will be prepared by a designated rapporteur in accordance with institutional guidelines.

WORKSHOP OBJECTIVES

This workshop was designed to identify the key questions that need to be addressed as a field to develop tractable biomarkers of neuroinflammation to assess disease progression or therapeutic efficacy, and thus to advance the development of therapeutics, said Linda Brady, director of the Division of Neuroscience and Basic Behavioral Science at the National Institute of Mental Health (NIMH). Brian Campbell, vice president of pharmacology at MindImmune Therapeutics, Inc., and George & Anne Ryan Research Professor of Neuroscience at The University of Rhode Island, gave examples of some questions. What are the unique features of neuroinflammation in acute versus chronic disease states? Are there different phenotypes that are important to measure in those conditions? What are the needs for biomarkers in acute versus chronic settings?

ORGANIZATION OF THE PROCEEDINGS

The following proceedings summarize the workshop presentations and discussions. Chapter 2 provides a summary of the myriad challenges to developing biomarkers of neuroinflammation as well as opportunities to address these challenges, as detailed in later chapters. Chapter 3 provides a primer on the mechanisms and manifestations of neuroinflammation across the acute to chronic neuroinflammation continuum. These mechanisms are further explored in Chapter 4, using as examples MS, traumatic brain injury (TBI), Huntington's disease (HD), Alzheimer's disease (AD), and neuropsychiatric disorders such as depression. Chapters 5 and 6 discuss neuroimaging biomarkers and fluid biomarkers of neuroinflammation, respectively. Chapter 7 offers the concluding thoughts of workshop participants on the challenges that still need to be addressed, and discusses ongoing efforts to build the collaborations to consolidate the data and expertise that will be needed to facilitate development and validation of neuroinflammatory biomarkers and to accelerate the development of new therapies.

2

Biomarkers of Neuroinflammation: Challenges and Potential Opportunities

Neuroinflammation is a pathological feature of a wide range of central nervous system (CNS) diseases, including classic neuroinflammatory disorders, such as multiple sclerosis (MS); neurodegenerative diseases, such as Alzheimer's disease (AD) and Huntington's disease (HD); disorders induced by brain injury; and neuropsychiatric disorders, such as depression and schizophrenia. Brian Campbell said that similar cell types and inflammatory mediators are induced across the range of these disorders, yet the consequences vary from toxic processes, such as the release of proinflammatory cytokines or reactive oxygen species, to reparative processes, such as the release of anti-inflammatory cytokines or stimulation of neuroprotective and angiogenic factors. These inflammatory mediators and other cellular markers could all potentially represent biomarkers of neuroinflammation, which in turn could be used to elucidate mechanisms, suggested Campbell. However, many workshop participants cited challenges that have hindered the development of such biomarkers. They also cited innovative approaches and collaborative efforts that are seeking to overcome these challenges.

OVERVIEW OF CHALLENGES

The Complex Biology of Neuroinflammation

Campbell described a neuroinflammatory process that is highly complex in terms of the activation of microglia, which are the resident immune cells of the brain; the cellular microenvironment, which includes not only microglia, but also astrocytes, oligodendrocytes, and peripherally derived immune cells; and the temporal correlation between different activation states of cells and disease phenotypes. In the absence of disease, neuroinflammatory and immune cells help maintain homeostasis, said Campbell. Amit Bar-Or, professor of neurology at the University of Pennsylvania, added that there is currently no comprehensive, functional immune profiling of the normal state on which diseases are superimposed. Added to this complexity is a limited understanding of the basic biology of microglia as they transition from resting to activated states and the completely unexplored role of the microbiota on microglial biology, said Gary Landreth, professor of anatomy and cell biology at the Stark Institute, Indiana University School of Medicine. The role that T cells play in neuroinflammatory diseases, including neuropsychiatric diseases, is also limited, despite the fact that T cells are known to play a major role in neuronal integrity, added Andrew Miller, William P. Timmie Professor of Psychiatry and Behavioral Sciences at the Emory University School of Medicine.

The complexity of neuroinflammation is exacerbated by substantial biological heterogeneity across individuals and over the disease course, including differences in the subsets of immune cells activated, said Campbell. Heterogeneity is seen not only in the types of cells but in their spatial and temporal appearance and functional activity states during development in healthy individuals as well as in normal aging and disease, added Linda Brady. She cited several aspects of neuroinflammation where a more detailed understanding is needed: (1) the response of immune cells and endothelial cells to the local microenvironment, (2) localized inflammatory responses, (3) the range of phenotypes in functional activity states of microglia and immune cells in normal and non-disease tissue over the life span of development, (4) the role of acute and chronic inflammation in homeostasis and disease states, and (5) under what conditions neuroinflammation has positive versus negative effects.

Given the complexity of neuroinflammation across the acute to chronic continuum in different diseases, different strategies may be needed to develop biomarkers that will both elucidate the pathophysiology of disease and be useful for therapeutic development purposes, said Edward Bullmore, who heads the Department of Psychiatry at the University of Cambridge and the Clinical Unit for GlaxoSmithKline in Cambridge. He added that there is also likely to be a need for more attention to statistical methods and computational tools, including novel tools to analyze high-dimensional data.

Exploring the Need for Better Biomarkers

Although some positron emission tomography (PET) ligands are available that recognize a neuroinflammatory signal, markers are not currently available to characterize different activation states of microglia, nor the consequences of microglia activation, such as whether they become more phagocytic, said Beth Stevens, associate professor of neurology at Harvard University Medical School; Boston Children's Hospital. PET ligands are also available to assess synaptic density, but Stevens said there is an urgent need for biomarkers of synaptic dysfunction, which could be particularly valuable for neuropsychiatric disorders where the affected circuits are not known. Markers of synaptic dysfunction not only could help identify those circuits and profile the normal condition and region-specific heterogeneity but could also provide information about when those circuits are affected, said Stevens. Biomarkers are also needed to identify regional variation in blood–brain barrier (BBB) dysfunction, added Richard Daneman, assistant professor of neuroscience and pharmacology at University of California, San Diego.

Campbell questioned whether any of the existing imaging biomarkers have adequate sensitivity in diseases where neuroinflammatory changes are subtle, such as depression, or to discriminate subpopulations and their changing microenvironments in diseases such as AD. Even when biomarkers are available, their relationship to disease course is unclear, said Bullmore, noting that cytokines and gene transcripts have been associated with CNS diseases, including depression, but association does not necessarily mean causation. He said this explanatory gap needs to be filled with mechanistic studies. In addition, longitudinal studies that look at a broad range of risks and phenotypes over time in relation to the emergence of depression and changes in peripheral biomarkers of inflammation could provide further information on the mechanisms involved, he said.

An audience participant noted that because neuroinflammation can produce both damaging and compensatory effects, it is critical to understand both the normal trajectory of pro- and anti-inflammatory molecules and signaling mechanisms as well as the extent to which activation of microglia and other immune cells represents a compensatory mechanism in a disease process. Miller suggested that researchers investigate under what conditions increased expression of these molecules reflect neuroinflammation versus normal physiological processes, such as synaptic plasticity.

Plasma-based peripheral biomarkers of inflammation would be less expensive, less invasive, and more accessible than central biomarkers measured in the cerebrospinal fluid (CSF) or through neuroimaging approaches, although central biomarkers may be closer to the disease site, said Bullmore. However, he added that resolving the tradeoff between these two approaches will require more data to make comparisons and establish links between the peripheral and central compartments.

Using Appropriate Animal Models

Animal models are widely used to study neuroinflammation, yet have limitations with regard to biomarker development. For example, Bar-Or said that, while animal modeling in MS has elucidated some important principles of immune regulation, trafficking, and neuronal interactions, there is no animal that develops actual MS, posing a challenge to elucidating certain pathophysiological aspects and developing targeted therapies.

Fiona Crawford, president and chief executive officer of the Roskamp Institute, described many animal models that have been explored to study traumatic brain injury (TBI). These models vary in terms of the genetic strain as well as by variations in the way the injury is induced. Mouse models have several advantages, including their accelerated life span and the availability of different strains of genetically manipulated animals. Nevertheless, while all of the preclinical models of TBI and human cases demonstrate inflammation, rodent models cannot show the hallmark chronic traumatic encephalopathy pathology of tau in the depths of the sulci, said Crawford. However, they do show other pathological features, including axonal transport issues, the presence of amyloid precursor protein, myelin loss, astrogliosis, and inflammation microgliosis, and they also show behavioral manifestations, such as decline in memory performance.

OVERVIEW OF POTENTIAL OPPORTUNITIES

Developing Static and Dynamic Biomarkers in Parallel

In the context of therapeutic development, biomarkers are needed for multiple purposes: to diagnose disease, monitor therapy, and demonstrate target engagement in clinical trials. Bar-Or proposed an onion-peel model

CHALLENGES AND POTENTIAL OPPORTUNITIES

of biomarker development (see Figure 2-1), in which more broadly applicable "static" biomarkers assessed with more easily accessible samples and technologies may be implemented in all cohort participants, while additional less accessible but potentially more disease-relevant "dynamic" biomarkers are developed in subsets of the cohort where practical. Intermediate biomarkers, such as those obtained from "omics" studies applied to easily accessible samples, can help generate hypotheses that guide dynamic biomarker development, he said.

Bullmore suggested that in clinical trials for anti-inflammatory drugs in non-psychiatric disorders, much earlier end point measurements of brain function and mental state changes should be adopted. If strong evidence could be generated showing that an anticytokine treatment had effects on brain function and mental state that preceded its effects on physical health, this would provide clear evidence of a mechanistically specific event, he said.

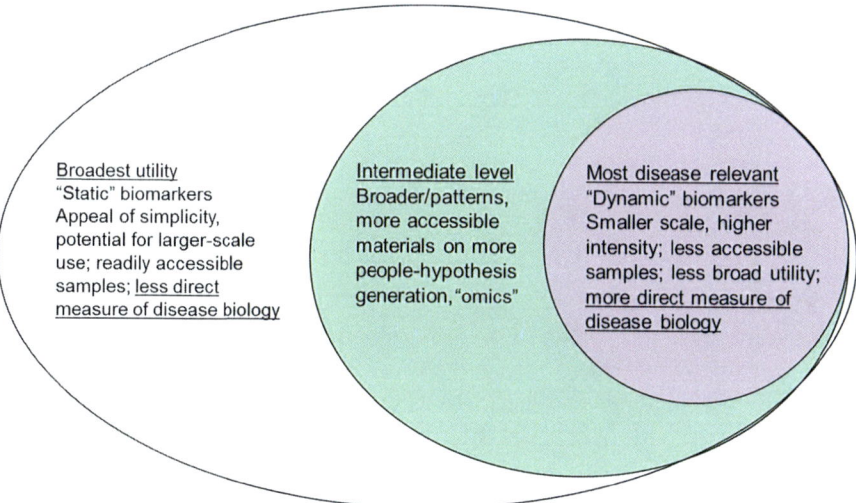

FIGURE 2-1 Onion-peel model of biomarker development. Both static and dynamic biomarkers may have value and should be developed in parallel, iteratively, and with one guiding the other.
SOURCE: Presentation by Bar-Or, March 21, 2017.

Developing Both Central and Peripheral Biomarkers

In terms of biomarker development for neuropsychiatric diseases where peripheral inflammation appears to play a role, Bullmore advocated for transcriptional or functional rather than cytokine assays because there is so much variability in cytokines and proteins in the peripheral blood. However, Miller noted that in non-neuropsychiatric inflammatory diseases, including cardiovascular disease, a protein marker called C-reactive protein (CRP) has proven to be a very strong predictor of disease development and also maps to changes in the brain. Bullmore said that focusing on the peripheral immune system increases the potential availability of biomarkers to guide the selection of patients and assess efficacy, which would reduce the risk of expensive late-stage clinical trial failures that have plagued CNS drug development. An audience participant added that peripheral biomarkers could provide better understanding of the dialogue between the brain and the immune system, for example, how exercise and environmental enrichment may impact depression.

Developing Novel Biomarkers of Neuroinflammation

While many neuroinflammatory mediators have been identified and are being developed as potential biomarkers, additional novel markers are emerging as understanding of the complex mechanisms involved becomes more refined. Stevens suggested that profiling proteomic and ribonucleic acid (RNA) sequencing in microglia and other cell players in affected versus non-affected brain regions over time could enable identification of novel sets of markers that could tell researchers more about function. She is currently collaborating with Steven McCarroll, director of genetics for the Broad Institute's Stanley Center for Psychiatric Research, to develop a molecular fingerprint of changes that occur in microglia from patients with HD and other diseases using the novel Drop-seq technology developed in his lab. Drop-seq allows for the study of cells in ways not previously possible, noted Landreth. Bullmore added that it could potentially be applied to thousands of cells obtained in a clean CSF tap to characterize phenotypes of cells close to the brain.

Other suggestions for potentially novel biomarkers include

- New PET ligands or imaging markers that could provide more information about microglia function and synaptic dysfunction (Stevens).

- Biomarkers obtained by examining both soluble phase and cell-based compartments, using tools that can be validly applied and validated in carefully cryo-preserved samples (Bar-Or).
- Biomarkers obtained by activating live cells to bring out disease-related and treatment-related differences (Bar-Or).
- Biomarkers obtained to test BBB disruption, activation of coagulation, and vascular alternations (Akassoglou, Daneman).

New Strategies for Biomarker Development

Given the complex mechanisms of neuroinflammation and its involvement in both healthy and disease states, many workshop participants stated that new strategies are needed to collect and analyze relevant data for biomarker development. Among the suggestions noted by individual workshop participants were:

- Steven Hyman, director of the Stanley Center for Psychiatric Research at the Broad Institute of Massachusetts Institute of Technology (MIT) and Harvard University, commented on the importance of collecting normative data for CSF markers, suggesting that understanding of many CNS disorders could be advanced substantially if serial CSF draws could be obtained from a normative developmental cohort.
- For neuropsychiatric diseases, Miller suggested subgrouping patients and looking at their responses to different treatment paradigms.
- Richard Perrin, assistant professor of neuropathology at the Washington University School of Medicine, noted that because aberrant synaptic pruning is common to all neurodegenerative diseases and probably psychiatric diseases that are not considered neurodegenerative, it will be important to learn from all of these diseases and use assays across disease fields.
- Bar-Or commented on the need for an iterative process, using animal and human studies to inform each other, rather than a siloed approach.
- Bullmore commented that because immunotherapeutics now comprise a large proportion of drugs in development for oncology and other disease areas, there is potential to leverage existing expertise, facilities, and molecules, and/or repurpose immunotherapy drugs already on the market for the treatment of CNS diseases.

- Because there appear to be links between inflammatory mediators and depression, Bullmore suggested that future clinical trials of anti-inflammatory drugs for non-psychiatric disorders include brain function and mental-stage changes, in addition to biomarkers of inflammation.
- Miles Herkenham, chief of the Section on Functional Neuroanatomy at the National Institute of Mental Health (NIMH), suggested that lymphocyte profiling might also represent a useful biomarker because the adaptive immune system has been shown to affect mood and, in animals, to improve hippocampal neurogenesis, which may be relevant in depression.
- Although several workshop participants spoke about the limited funding currently available for research on neuroinflammatory diseases, one audience participant commented that funding is available through the Department of Defense for Gulf War illness research, including research related to TBI.

Collaborative Approaches for Biomarker Development

Several workshop participants mentioned frequently that collaboration was a necessary strategy to advance the development of neuroinflammation biomarkers. For example, Stevens advocated for building mechanisms to bring people together to collaborate and share samples, expertise, and data. While collaborations are discussed further in Chapter 7, some of the specific examples cited include the following:

- William Potter, senior advisor to the director at NIMH, noted the benefits of integrating studies conducted across stages of disease and across species. Stevens added that this approach may require a consortium, picking out three or four target mechanisms and looking at them from different perspectives and areas of expertise in multiple animal models and humans.
- Katerina Akassoglou, senior investigator at the Gladstone Institute of Neurological Disease, University of California, San Francisco (UCSF), suggested conducting longitudinal studies in large, well-defined patient populations, such as the Expression, Proteomics, Imaging, Clinical (EPIC) MS cohort at UCSF.[1] This

---

[1] For more information see http://msepicstudy.com/epic (accessed July 17, 2017).

cohort includes primary and secondary progressive MS patients at multiple time points.
- McCarroll proposed a definitive experiment to look at the relationship between cell-type-specific RNA expression and imaging data levels for TSPO (translocator protein) or other putative markers of neuroinflammation in order to determine the true cellular sources of these biomarkers. Tarek Samad, head of neurodegeneration at Pfizer Inc., and Perrin advocated for expanding this approach beyond TSPO.
- McCarroll also suggested collaborations to apply Drop-seq technology to better understand the full set of cellular and molecular events in disease states, including which cells produce particular biomarkers, and how the expression of these markers varies among patients. He added that due to ongoing innovations in the Drop-seq technology, such experiments are now possible whenever archival, fresh-frozen brain samples have been saved.
- Perrin said biospecimens from the Knight Alzheimer's Disease Research Center (ADRC) at Washington University are available for appropriate studies. He said that although tissue from the hippocampus is limited because of its small size in humans, tissue from other brain areas is more readily available.
- Because subject recruitment presents a major challenge to evaluating PET ligands in depression and AD, Robert Innis, chief of the Molecular Imaging Branch at NIMH, offered to work with investigators in this area by providing free PET scans at NIMH facilities to patients in whom plasma and CSF biomarkers have been assessed.

3

State of the Science of Neuroinflammation in Central Nervous System Disorders

Highlights

- Microglia are the resident immune cells of the central nervous system (CNS); however, there is more to neuroinflammation than microglia (Campbell) and there is still much to learn about microglial biology (Innis, Landreth).
- The primary function of microglia is homeostasis, but they also have other functions, including surveilling the brain for perturbations, pruning synapses, and modulating neural systems and circuits (Campbell).
- The observation that receptors such as TSPO (translocator protein) and TREM2 (triggering receptor expressed on myeloid cells 2), and other proteins, such as Iba1 expressed by microglia, are upregulated in almost all CNS disorders indicates that activation of microglia plays a prominent role in diseases of the brain (Campbell).
- While synaptic pruning is a normal developmental process, aberrant synaptic pruning may underlie many neurological, neurodevelopmental, and neuropsychiatric diseases, including schizophrenia and autism as well as diseases of aging (Stevens).
- Identifying the signals involved in synaptic pruning may unveil biomarkers and therapeutic targets for many CNS diseases (Stevens).
- Blood–brain barrier (BBB) dysfunction is common in many neuroinflammatory CNS diseases, including stroke, brain trauma, epilepsy, and multiple sclerosis (MS), possibly through common genetic and molecular mechanisms, which may be possible to exploit for the identification of biomarkers and therapeutics (Daneman).
- Fibrinogen, a blood protein involved in coagulation, is also involved in activating neuroinflammation and neurodegeneration and is important for communication between the peripheral immune system and the CNS (Akassoglou).

NOTE: These points were made by the individual speakers identified above; they are not intended to reflect a consensus among workshop participants.

Neuroinflammation is similar to peripheral inflammation in many respects and in at least some prototypical neuroinflammatory diseases, such as MS, in which similar types of immune cells are sequestered into regions of damage, said Brian Campbell. He described inflammation as a response by the immune system to either segregate or remove a damaging stimulus in order to help facilitate the healing process by increasing blood vessel permeability, recruiting immune cells into the area, and releasing inflammatory mediators, such as cytokines and chemokines. In the CNS, the resident immune cells are microglia, which can be detected via positron emission tomography (PET) imaging with ligands that bind to the TSPO, also known as the peripheral benzodiazepine receptor (PBR). In MS, elevated TSPO binding is seen in both the acute and chronic inflammatory states (Ciccarelli et al., 2014) and is also seen in other CNS diseases such as Alzheimer's disease (AD), Huntington's disease (HD), Parkinson's disease (PD), and stroke, diseases that Campbell noted are not classically considered neuroinflammatory conditions. However, Gary Landreth commented that neuroinflammation is an invariant feature of neurodegenerative disease. Despite the fact that there are hundreds of publications linking TSPO to neuroinflammatory disease, Campbell said there is more to neuroinflammation than microglia, and Robert Innis said much remains unknown about microglial biology.

MICROGLIA AND NEUROINFLAMMATION

Microglia comprise approximately 10 percent of cells in the brain, said Campbell. They derive exclusively from yolk sac progenitors, not from bone marrow or other hematopoietic stem cells, and enter the brain very early in development, according to Beth Stevens. Landreth added that all microglia derive from cell proliferation and self-renewal of these progenitors, but said that the biology around these progenitors and the natural history of microglia, including metabolic changes, have been poorly explored. Similar to the way peripheral immune cells function, microglia defend against damage by continuously surveilling the brain for perturbations. But Campbell said they also modulate neural systems and circuits, provide trophic support, and cause synapse pruning (see Figure 3-1). Indeed, he said that the basic function of microglia is homeostasis. Stevens noted that microglia appear to undergo dramatic changes in the context of normal aging, increasing classic immune responses, but decreasing some of their homeostatic sensing functions. She said they also

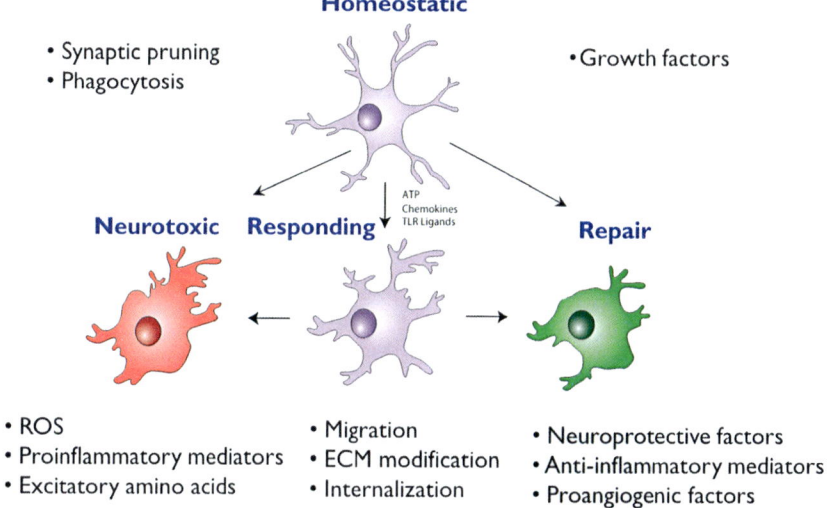

FIGURE 3-1 Microglia serve multiple functions in the brain, including synaptic pruning, phagocytosis, and the secretion of growth factors to maintain homeostasis. When activated they may become neurotoxic or reparative.
NOTE: ATP = adenosine triphosphate; ECM = extracellular matrix; ROS = reactive oxygen species; TLR = toll-like receptor.
SOURCE: Presentation by Campbell, March 20, 2017.

interact with astrocytes, although the relationship between these two cell types and the effect on neuroinflammatory disease is not well understood. Landreth noted that in addition to resident microglia, an inflammatory subset of blood-borne monocytes infiltrates the brain in a number of CNS disorders, and then acquires microglia markers and produces inflammatory cytokines within 72 hours that make them indistinguishable from resident microglia (Sieweke and Allen, 2013).

Understanding the biology of neuroinflammation was advanced through studies of the rare, progressive neurodegenerative Nasu-Hakola disease (also known as PLOSL), which arises from mutations in the TREM2 gene (Bianchin et al., 2004), said Landreth. TREM2 is only expressed in myeloid cells (i.e., microglia in the brain), indicating that these cells are sufficient to drive neurodegeneration all by themselves, he said. Moreover, many genome-wide association studies (GWASs) have identified variants of TREM2 that increase the risk of AD and other neurodegenerative diseases. One variant in particular, R47H, is sufficient to increase the risk of AD threefold, an effect size similar to that observed for ApoEε4, said Landreth (Guerreiro et al., 2013).

In AD, the TREM2-positive inflammatory cells surrounding plaques have been shown to be peripherally derived monocytes rather than resident microglia, and knocking out TREM2 in AD mouse models largely abrogates the accumulation of inflammatory cells around the plaques in an age- and disease-progression–dependent fashion (Jay et al., 2015). Yet, while TREM2 has become the focus of research on neuroinflammation, Landreth said there remains a poor understanding of the biology, including the differential biology of the resident microglia and infiltrating monocytes over the course of the disease, and the consequences of different mutations.

TREM2 also appears to affect neuroinflammation through soluble extracellular fragments shed through cleavage of the cell-surface receptor. A recent paper showed that these cleavage products interact with microglia to drive a strong proinflammatory response (Zhong et al., 2017). In addition, elevations of soluble TREM2 in the cerebrospinal fluid have been shown to correlate with the deposition of amyloid in patients with dominantly inherited forms of AD (Suarez-Calvet et al., 2016), suggesting that soluble forms of TREM2 may represent a valuable biomarker for disease, said Landreth.

While the TSPO and TREM2 research supports the view that microglial activation is important in nearly all CNS disorders, Campbell noted that an operational definition of microglial activation is still needed. He said that when stimulated, microglia enter a responding stage with a number of different phenotypes that may alternatively internalize toxic substances, take on a migratory phenotype, release proinflammatory cytokines or reactive oxygen species, or release factors involved in repairing, such as neuroprotective or angiogenic factors, anti-inflammatory cytokines, prostaglandins, microvesicles, and microRNAs or miRNAs (Loane and Byrnes, 2010). Biomarkers to identify these different phenotypes could advance understanding about not just what causes microglia to become activated but also the consequences of that activation, said Campbell. They could also help define the temporal correlation between different activation states of microglia in different diseases and patient populations, he said. Fiona Crawford concurred, noting that microglia are very fluid, changing their presentation depending on the context and the other cells they are interacting with at any given moment. Mouse models could prove very useful in understanding microglial activation profiles that reflect biological processes in vulnerable versus non-vulnerable regions of the brain, added Stevens. For example, her lab has shown in both HD and AD mouse models that changes in microglia markers in early stages of disease are very different from those seen once inflammation begins.

Landreth mentioned work by Joseph El Khoury and colleagues in which they identified a "microglial sensome," a panel of microglial-specific genes that may be up- or downregulated in aging and various CNS diseases, and thus may be useful in identifying biomarkers (Hickman et al., 2013). Amit Bar-Or added that the complex nature of microglial biology and the lack of clarity about whether changes from normal are harmful or beneficial has stymied efforts to develop useful biomarkers.

SYNAPTIC PRUNING

As mentioned earlier, microglial function goes beyond neuroinflammation. Microglia also sculpt and prune neural circuits during normal development. This process is highly regulated and not random with respect to when and which synapses are removed, and the fact that this is developmentally regulated suggests that there must be both "on" and "off" signals, said Stevens. Moreover, synaptic pruning is necessary for precise synaptic connectivity and brain wiring, she said. The normal pruning process becomes aberrantly regulated in a host of different neurological diseases, contributing to synapse loss and dysfunction, said Stevens, adding that defects in pruning or remodeling may underlie neurological, neurodevelopmental, and neuropsychiatric disorders, including schizophrenia and autism, as well as in diseases of aging, such as AD. Synapse loss in AD appears to occur at an early stage of the disease, before overt inflammation, and is correlated to cognitive dysfunction. This correlation is even stronger than the correlation between cognitive dysfunction and plaques and tangle pathology, said Stevens.

Stevens commented on whether there could be a common mechanism in these diverse diseases that tells microglia which synapses to prune. Specific synapses and circuits are known to be vulnerable in various diseases, she said, which could mean there are mechanisms regulating the recognition process that might be relevant in the context of these diseases. For example, she noted that while synapses with less active inputs tend to be selectively eliminated, how they signal microglia about differences in neuronal activity is not well understood. Stevens suggested that identifying these signals could yield therapeutic targets and/or biomarkers. Signals that appear important in this process are associated with the complement cascade, in particular C1q and a downstream component, C3, she said. She added that while the complement cascade is best understood in the context of immunity and the process of clearing pathogens from cells, complement components may similarly tag and clear less active synapses. Her lab and others are just beginning to tease out the steps, proteins, receptors, and protective signals involved in this process.

There is also evidence that the control mechanisms in this system may be lost in disease states, she said. For example, genetic evidence from Steve McCarroll's lab and others suggests that a particular form of C4 increases the risk of schizophrenia, possibly from overpruning of certain circuits. In neurodegenerative disease, pathways that normally are turned off may be turned back on again, suggesting a possible treatment target, said Stevens.

BLOOD–BRAIN BARRIER DYSFUNCTION

The "blood–brain barrier" is a term used to describe unique properties of the CNS vasculature that prevent molecules and ions from going from the blood into the brain, according to Richard Daneman. It is critical to maintain brain homeostasis and to protect the CNS from toxins, pathogens, and even the body's own immune system; its importance is highlighted by diseases in which it is compromised, such as in stroke, brain trauma, epilepsy, and MS, said Daneman.

Most of the properties of the BBB are manifested within the endothelial cells that make up the walls of the blood vessels. Daneman described multiple differences among endothelial cells in the CNS compared to those in other tissues. First, CNS endothelial cells are held together by tight junctions. They also undergo extremely low rates of transcytosis or vesicle-mediated trafficking, and express proteins that pump out small lipophilic molecules that have gotten into the brain and selectively transport specific metabolites into the brain. Finally, they express low levels of molecules that in other tissues are responsible for binding immune cells to facilitate their entry into those tissues. All of these properties may be lost in the presence of neurological disease, said Daneman. He added that work done in the 1980s showed that these properties are not intrinsic to endothelial cells, but are induced by the CNS microenvironment. Understanding how the BBB breaks down in different diseases could lead to the identification of both biomarkers and treatment targets, he said.

Daneman's lab has studied the BBB in four disease models: stroke, MS, TBI, and epilepsy, each of which has a mouse model on which to conduct experimental studies. All of these diseases show massive BBB dysfunction at the site of the injury or lesion in both human and mouse models, he said. Yet while each has a different trigger—hypoxia/ischemia in stroke, inflammation in MS, trauma in TBI, and neural activity in epilepsy—Daneman and colleagues showed that the pattern of gene expression is similar over multiple time points corresponding to acute, subacute, and chronic responses. This allowed the researchers to identify a BBB dysfunction module—197 genes that are upregulated in at least three of the diseases, suggesting there may be a common pathway for BBB dysfunction. Daneman's team went on to classify these genes into three groups with different temporal patterns. One group peaks early in the disease and then goes down at later time points, while a second group peaks at the subacute time point when there is the most BBB dysfunction. The third group often peaks at the subacute time point, but in some diseases it persists on the blood vessels into the chronic phase for well over 1 month after the initial insult. Interestingly these 197 genes are normally expressed at low levels in brain endothelial cells, but at high levels in leakier peripheral endothelial cells of the heart, kidney, and lung, suggesting a mechanism for breach of the BBB, said Daneman.

The other cells that are important in BBB function are the pericytes, which sit outside the vessels. Earlier work by Daneman and colleagues showed that the BBB is leakier when there are fewer pericytes (Daneman et al., 2010). Moreover, pericyte-deficient mice showed an upregulation of 145 peripheral endothelial genes, but only 1 of 400 BBB-specific genes, suggesting that pericytes inhibit the expression of these leaky genes. These observations led Daneman to hypothesize that upregulation of peripheral endothelial genes leads to BBB disruption during disease, at least in part because of a loss of endothelial–pericyte interactions. A screen in his lab for candidate genes that disrupt cellular barriers led to the identification of a family of genes (the EHD family) that regulate endocytosis and vesicle trafficking, said Daneman. One member of this family—EHD4—is upregulated in stroke and MS animal models, that is, conditions associated with BBB dysfunction, he said. Moreover, his lab showed that mice engineered to express high levels of EHD4 also showed BBB dysfunction, including fibrinogen leakage. Taken together, these studies suggest there is a common molecular pathway across many different neurological diseases for BBB dysfunction, which is characterized by loss of endothelial–pericyte interactions, upregulation of endothelial genes, increased vesicle trafficking and disruption of tight junctions, and leakage through the pericellular barrier, said Daneman. Development of endothelial biomarkers could be used to identify the location of damage to the BBB as well as the location of past damage, he said, adding that there may also be the potential to use these molecules as guide posts for targeted delivery of therapeutics. Daneman's group is also working to identify serum biomarkers of BBB dysfunction by inducing breakdown of the BBB in an animal model and then analyzing serum with proteomic and metabolomic technologies.

Daneman noted that there are other possible mechanisms for moving cells and antibodies into the CNS, for example, different types of endothelial cells in the meningeal or choroid plexus vessels, antibody transporters at the BBB, the glymphatic system, and the meningeal lymphatic system. Edward Bullmore added that not all parts of the BBB are equally impermeable and that there may be active transport mechanisms for some immune modulators, such as interleukin 6 (IL-6).

FIBRINOGEN AND THE NEUROVASCULAR INTERFACE

Katerina Akassoglou has been studying the consequences of BBB disruption in diseases such as MS, stroke, and brain trauma, and classic neurodegenerative conditions, such as AD. Epidemiological studies show that increased leakage of plasma proteins from inside the vessels to the surrounding tissue correlates with worsening pathology and worse prognosis, she said. Her lab aims to identify the peripheral triggers and molecular determinants of this pathological process, which could lead not only to the development of new imaging tools to image the neurovascular interface but also to new therapeutics, animal models, and biomarkers. In particular, they focus on fibrinogen, a protein that is abundantly deposited in human neurological diseases as well as in animal models; that plays dual functions in both blood coagulation and inflammation; and that represents a druggable interaction.

Fibrinogen is a non-pathogenic soluble protein in the blood, but with the action of thrombin, it forms insoluble fibrin that binds to platelets to form clots and is highly proinflammatory, said Akassoglou. She and others have shown that fibrin is required for the development of many CNS diseases, including MS (Adams et al., 2007; Davalos et al., 2012), brain trauma (Schachtrup et al., 2010), and AD (Cortes-Canteli et al., 2010). Akassoglou and her colleagues hypothesized that two non-overlapping epitopes in the fibrinogen molecule mediate coagulation and inflammation, and wondered if these two activities could be disassociated either genetically or pharmacologically to target the damaging function in inflammation without affecting beneficial effects in hemostasis. What they found is that microglia are the main cell targets of fibrin in the CNS through the binding of one of these epitopes to the microglia CD11b/CD18 integrin receptor (complement receptor 3), while another epitope in the fibrin molecule binds to platelets to cause coagulation (Adams et al., 2007). Akassoglou said fibrinogen is specific among plasma proteins to induce microglia activation (Davalos et al., 2012). Fibrinogen induces demyelination and recruits macrophages and T cells (Ryu et al., 2015), she said, and blocking the interaction of fibrin and the CD11b receptor was shown in mouse models to suppress innate immunity and the downstream effects of neurodegeneration (Adams et al., 2007; Davalos et al., 2012). As described in Chapter 5, Akassoglou and colleagues are developing molecular probes to be used with magnetic resonance imaging to monitor coagulation activity in neuroinflammatory disease.

4

Neuroinflammation in Disease

Highlights

- Multiple sclerosis, the prototypical neuroinflammatory disease, involves an aberrant balance of T, B, and myeloid cell responses (potentially including microglia), all of which represent potential targets for biomarker development (Bar-Or).
- Traumatic brain injury (TBI), even in mild cases, triggers a complex disease process involving both innate and adaptive immune responses, including neuroinflammation (Crawford).
- Several different animal models have been particularly valuable to understand the pathophysiological mechanisms of TBI, and to study potential therapeutic strategies (Crawford).
- Animal models of Huntington's disease (HD) have been particularly valuable to study the role of microglia and the complement cascade in synapse loss, which is a central feature of neurodegenerative disease. These models suggest that synapse loss precedes overt inflammation (Stevens).
- Alzheimer's disease (AD) involves more than plaques and tangles, including neuroinflammation, synaptic and neuronal dysfunction, and cell death. The study of AD has led to the identification of many promising cerebrospinal fluid (CSF) and plasma biomarker candidates (Perrin).
- Biomarker studies suggest that peripheral immune and inflammatory mechanisms may play important roles in the pathogenesis of neuropsychiatric diseases, such as depression, although the pathways that link inflammation with these diseases is unclear (Bullmore).

NOTE: These points were made by the individual speakers identified above; they are not intended to reflect a consensus among workshop participants.

MULTIPLE SCLEROSIS

MS represents the prototypic neuroinflammatory disease and is a major cause of neurological disability in young adults, although highly variable and unpredictable. Amit Bar-Or noted that in the past decade, multiple treatment options have become available, which perturb the complex pathophysiology of MS in many ways. However, selecting the treatment modality that will be best suited for individual patients remains an ongoing challenge, he said. Biomarkers that allow characterization of relevant biologies in individual patients would allow clinicians to choose the most appropriate treatment (both efficacy and safety), monitor response to treatment, and possibly change or sequence treatments, said Bar-Or.

Bar-Or described a simplified immune pathogenesis model of MS in which immune cells in the periphery are activated, upregulating a series of molecules that enable the immune cells to more efficiently cross the blood–brain barrier (BBB), where they are reactivated. Historically, MS has been thought of as primarily a T-cell disease, but Bar-Or said that recent research shows that B cells are also important. Bar-Or said that to capture the complexity and heterogeneity of the disease, it will be necessary to measure the biologies of multiple different cell subsets. The mechanisms that underlie the aberrant balance of T, B, and myeloid cells may be a target for biomarker development, he said.

Indeed, the most recently approved treatment for MS—ocrelizumab—selectively targets B cells that express CD20, said Bar-Or. However, ocrelizumab treatment has no apparent impact on the levels of antibodies in CSF, suggesting that non-antibody functions of B cells are important (Hauser et al., 2017). Bar-Or and colleagues have shown that B cells produce different cytokines depending on the mode of activation. Compared to healthy controls, the B cells of MS patients produce increased proinflammatory cytokines and reduced levels of anti-inflammatory cytokines that regulate T-cell function and autoimmunity (Bar-Or et al.,

2010). They have also shown in patients with MS an increased number of B cells that produce granulocyte macrophage-colony stimulating factor (GM-CSF), a cytokine that activates myeloid cells to produce proinflammatory responses. B-cell depletion diminishes myeloid cell proinflammatory responses (Li et al., 2015). From a biomarker perspective, this means that measurement of these pro- and anti-inflammatory cytokines may enable definition of an individual's functional immune profile, said Bar-Or.

Magnetic resonance imaging (MRI) is a highly sensitive tool for diagnosing MS, demonstrating that the disease is dynamic, multifocal, and diffuse, said Bar-Or, adding that gadolinium enhancement further demonstrates a breach of integrity in the BBB, which is thought to represent perivascular inflammation. However, Bar-Or said that within the CNS compartment, damage extends beyond the white-matter focal areas captured by standard T2-weighted MR images to gray-matter areas, including areas at the surface of the cortex. Indeed, cortical pathology seems to correlate better than white-matter pathology with longer-term disability, cognitive dysfunction, and social issues that people with MS experience, he said. Histopathological studies have shown that immune cells accumulate at the meninges in individuals with MS, and of interest is whether they contribute to cortical injury. Within the cortext underlying such meningeal immune cell collections, there is evidence of neuronal injury and microglial activation. This microglial activation occurs in a graded pattern from the surface inward, suggesting that a secreted factor released from meningeal immune cells contributes to neuronal damage (Magliozzi et al., 2010). Bar-Or suggested that it may be possible to develop this factor as a biomarker.

Measurement of analytes in the CSF and serum provides complementary information, said Bar-Or. For example, oligoclonal bands and immunoglobulin G (IgG) in CSF enable a diagnosis of CNS neuroinflammatory disease. Serum biomarkers that may distinguish MS from other CNS inflammatory diseases include antibodies against aquaporin 4 (AQP4), which are diagnostic for neuromyelitis optica (NMO) spectrum disease, a condition that is pathologically distinct from MS and has different therapeutic implications, said Bar-Or. There is active interest in whether the presence of serum myelin oligodendrocyte glycoprotein (MOG)-directed antibodies may reflect a subtype of MS or another entity. Other blood biomarkers that may be measured when starting treatment or considering a change in treatment include interferon beta–neutralizing antibodies, anti-JC antibodies, lymphopenia, and B-cell counts, he said. He also mentioned many candidate biomarkers. Those that show the most promise include neurofilament in CSF and serum, chitinase 3 like 1 in CSF, and some miRNAs. The cooperativity of different cell types could also be assessed by simultaneously assessing levels of different biomarkers in those cell subsets. This would require a concerted investment in dynamic cell-based assays, but would provide a much-needed added layer to biomarker development efforts, said Bar-Or.

Indeed, despite the development of biomarkers that reveal important aspects of disease, substantial discrepancies remain among the time course of imaging markers, clinical disease, and biological progression represented by peripherally mediated and CNS-compartmentalized inflammatory injury, said Bar-Or.

Moreover, he said, the relationship between inflammation and degeneration remains unclear. He cited a recent small study of patients with poor-prognosis, early-stage, aggressive MS, which showed that complete immunoablation followed by autologous bone marrow transplantation essentially halted disease progression, suggesting that robustly removing peripheral inflammation prevented neuroinflammation and neurodegeneration (Atkins et al., 2016). Bone marrow transplantation has been unsuccessful in later-stage disease, when CNS-compartmentalized processes are acting relatively independently of peripherally mediated inflammation, said Bar-Or.

TRAUMATIC BRAIN INJURY

TBI is a major cause of death and disability that has recently attracted increased attention because of the wars in Iraq and Afghanistan and increased awareness of the negative consequences of sports injuries, said Fiona Crawford. The vast majority of military cases are mild, yet even these have significant health impacts. Chronic traumatic encephalopathy (CTE), such as that seen in boxers, football players, and other athletes, represents a subset of TBI with a distinctive presentation that may include marked behavioral changes, she said, adding that TBI is also known to be a risk factor for AD in later life or other neurodegenerative diseases.

Crawford described the complex disease processes underlying both the acute injury and the secondary consequences of TBI, including calcium dysregulation, mitochondrial dysfunction, free radical generation, and neuroinflammation. Both innate and adaptive immune responses are invoked with the production of many cytokines and chemokines, the recruitment of T lymphocytes, and the activation of microglia, she said. Following the acute injury, these responses represent attempts to repair damage, said Crawford, and the persistence of the negative consequences of microglial activation causes chronic problems. The timing of these responses is important in order to identify the correct therapeutic window, said Crawford. Although many compounds have shown positive effects in preclinical rodent models, translation to human populations has been unsuccessful, which she said may be explained by the complexity and heterogeneity of these responses in humans.

Crawford advocated for increased attention in the preclinical space to better model the consequences of TBI. She described an array of animal models that have been developed that differ in terms of the animals used and the type of injury induced. She noted that mice have the advantage of being cheap, are available in many genetically manipulated strains, and have a life span that allows for relatively short studies. However, she also cited challenges associated with using animal models. For example, there are major differences in the brain architecture between mouse and human, and mice do not develop the hallmark pathology for CTE that is seen in humans—deposition of tau in the depths of the sulci—although she said that many other pathological features are similar across species. Crawford and colleagues have demonstrated in their mouse models similar axonal transport changes and axonal injury, accumulation of amyloid precursor protein (APP), myelin loss, astrogliosis, and inflammation microgliosis. Pigs have also been used in rotational models, she said.

Much of Crawford's early work used a controlled cortical impact (CCI) model, which involves a craniectomy and produces a relatively severe injury. There are also blast injury, fluid percussion, and rotational models. The one common denominator in all of these models is neuroinflammation, said Crawford.

More recently, she and her colleagues have developed a closed-head-injury model of mild TBI, where they can test single or repetitive injury compared to sham injury, with no fracture or bleeding. Using this model, they showed that the mice perform poorly on neurobehavioral testing and demonstrate progressive and life-long changes in microgliosis (which they visualize histopathologically by Iba1 binding), astrocytosis (GFAP binding), and inflammation (phospho-STAT3 binding) in mice after repetitive mild TBI (r-mTBI–5 hits over 9 days) compared to sham controls (Mouzon et al., 2012, 2014). They also used this model to test whether targeting neuroinflammation with a compound called anatabine—which has shown efficacy in mouse models of AD, MS, and tauopathy—ameliorated the problems. In the r-mTBI model, anatabine had minimal acute effects, but dramatically improved performance on neurobehavioral testing 6 months after injury, reduced Iba1 staining in the hippocampus and corpus callosum at 9 months after injury, and reduced GFAP staining in the hippocampus, said Crawford. Anatabine reduced microgliosis and astrocytosis even when first administered 9 months after injury, suggesting a large therapeutic window, she said. However, when anatabine treatment was discontinued after 9 months, neuroinflammation appeared to reemerge, suggesting that anatabine suppressed but did not eradicate the damage (Ferguson et al., 2017). Crawford suggested that an adaptive response or epigenetic mechanism might explain this phenomenon. Indeed, she noted that posttraumatic stress disorder (PTSD) often occurs in combination with TBI, and that the sleep disturbances that characterize PTSD are thought to influence epigenetic changes.

Tau pathology persisting after the cessation of injuries has been particularly difficult to recapitulate in TBI mouse models. Using the same mild injury in a new paradigm of two hits per week over 3 months, Crawford and colleagues have demonstrated persistence of tau pathology at 3 months after injury. Crawford and colleagues suggested that the tau phenotype emerges only in the presence of concomitant neuroinflammation. This may indicate that phosphorylation of tau at the beginning of injury is a positive response, but that persistent hyperphosphorylation only happens in the inflamed environment, said Crawford.

HUNTINGTON'S DISEASE

Beth Stevens described her work to understand the mechanisms underlying neurodegenerative diseases by studying HD, the most common autosomal dominant, monogenetic neurodegenerative disease, which is characterized by disorders of movement, cognition, and behavior. The mutation that causes HD is an expansion of cytosine-adenosine-guanine (CAG) repeats in the gene for huntingtin protein, said Stevens, noting that although the mutation occurs in all cells in the body, there is a selective vulnerability to neurodegeneration of the neural circuit between the motor cortex and striatum, and medium spiny neurons in the striatum. This regional and cellular specificity and the availability of several mouse models make HD a useful model to examine the mechanisms underlying synapse loss, said Stevens. Because the presence of the mutation can be used to identify individuals who will develop HD, Stevens's lab has also been able to study synaptic loss in the earliest stages of disease in human tissue through a collaboration with Richard Faull from the University of Auckland, who operates a large HD brain bank in New Zealand. These studies show that progressive synapse loss begins in a regionally specific manner in disease and in the absence of neuroinflammation. In animal models, they have been able to follow synapse loss over time, demonstrating that it begins early in the preclinical stages of disease, even before there is overt inflammation.

Stevens's lab has also been investigating the role of microglia and components of the complement cascade in synaptic loss. They have demonstrated a striking increase in two markers for complement—C1q and C3—in vulnerable brain regions in HD mice compared to wildtype, with deposition at the vulnerable synapses. In human tissue, they have also shown an upregulation in complement proteins in the HD brain. Using microglial stains, they have also shown a dramatic change in microglia in vulnerable regions of the mouse brain. However, to better understand functional impairments in microglia, Stevens said that novel biomarkers are needed. She has been working with Steve McCarroll to profile the proteome and RNA transcriptome of microglia in affected versus non-affected brain regions to try to create a molecular fingerprint of changes that occur. McCarroll's approach is discussed in more detail in Chapter 6.

ALZHEIMER'S DISEASE

The brain pathology that eventually leads to dementia in people with AD starts early, when people are still cognitively normal, said Richard Perrin. He noted that the amyloid cascade hypothesis, which has been the basis of most treatments in development, posits that the deposition of amyloid plaques is the first pathological feature, followed by the accumulation of neurofibrillary tangles, with neuronal integrity declining along the way (Perrin et al., 2009). However, Perrin emphasized that there is more to AD than plaques and tangles, including neuroinflammation, synaptic and neuronal dysfunction, and cell death (Fagan and Perrin, 2012) (see Figure 4-1). Recognition of the complex pathological

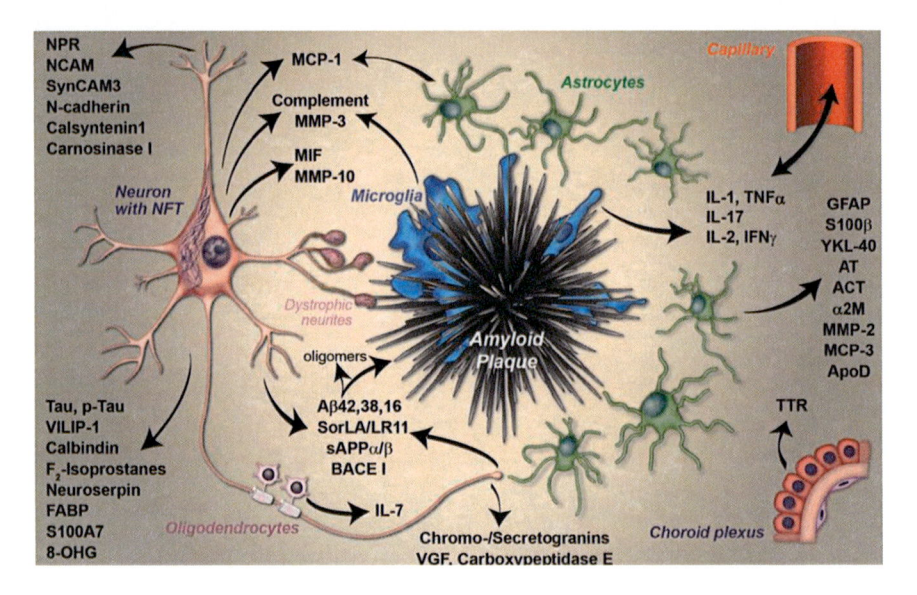

FIGURE 4-1 Although amyloid plaques may be the core pathological feature of Alzheimer's disease, many other processes contribute to neuronal injury and neurodegeneration, including different subsets of neuroinflammatory molecules produced by neurons, microglia, and astrocytes.
SOURCES: Presentation by Perrin, March 21, 2017; Fagan and Perrin, 2012.

processes that result in AD has given rise to a large number of promising CSF and plasma biomarker candidates. Indeed, study of these biomarkers has provided information about disease pathogenesis, said Perrin. For example, they show that brain amyloid is preceded by peripheral inflammation and low insulin signaling and that it coincides with low adiposity, low insulin signaling, and an anti-inflammatory milieu. Amyloid-associated dementia is also preceded by neuroinflammation as well as vasculopathy and BBB dysfunction and other hormonal and metabolic changes. Many of these pathophysiological changes may represent targets for therapy, said Perrin. His research to identify these novel CSF biomarkers is discussed further in Chapter 6.

IMMUNOPSYCHIATRY

Mental health disorders are the number one global cause of disability-adjusted life years, yet investment is disproportionately low, said Edward Bullmore. He suggested that innovation in drug development for neuropsychiatric disorders will require a pivot away from the focus on targets expressed in the brain, such as neurotransmitter receptors or transporters, in favor of targets in the peripheral immune system. Indeed, he noted that while 30 years ago the brain and immune system were thought to be strictly segregated from one another by the BBB, it is now recognized that there is physiological and therapeutically tractable cross-talk between the brain and immune system through the vagal inflammatory reflex (Tracey, 2002). Moreover, Bullmore said there is a strong reason to believe that immune or inflammatory mechanisms are involved in the pathogenesis of neuropsychiatric diseases. He argued that focusing on the peripheral immune system increases the potential availability of biomarkers to guide the selection of patients and assess efficacy, which would reduce the risk of expensive late-stage clinical trial failures that have plagued CNS drug development. Furthermore, because immunotherapeutics now make up a large proportion of drugs in development for oncology and other diseases, there is the potential to leverage existing expertise, facilities, and molecules, and/or repurpose drugs already on the market, said Bullmore (Bullmore and Lynall, 2014).

Bullmore noted that the role of inflammation in depression, and the potential usefulness of inflammatory biomarkers, was supported by a cumulative meta-analysis of studies over the past 20 years that showed a moderately strong and robust association between major depressive disorder (MDD) and the proinflammatory cytokines interleukin 6 (IL-6) and C-reactive protein (CRP) (Haapakoski et al., 2015). In a more recent study conducted by a consortium that Bullmore leads, which was funded by the Medical Research Council (MRC) (see Chapter 7), analysis of microarray data from earlier studies yielded a list of genes that were over- and underexpressed in depression, and showed—through an ontogeny analysis—that overexpressed genes were enriched for innate immune functions while underexpressed genes were enriched for adaptive immune functions.

Several studies have also provided evidence indicating that these markers of inflammation reflect causative mechanisms in depression, said Bullmore. For example, in a study conducted in a birth cohort population from Avon County, England, IL-6 and CRP levels obtained at 9 years of age were shown to be associated with an increased risk of developing depression at age 18 (Khandaker et al., 2014). Similarly, Bullmore cited unpublished data from the MRC Consortium showing that elevated CRP levels in non-depressed women in 2004 and 2008 were associated with approximately a threefold increased risk of becoming depressed in 2012, compared to women with no evidence of inflammation.

Identifying what the causative mechanisms are that link inflammation to depression remains a substantial gap in the literature; although a few studies have been done, said Bullmore. In one study, typhoid vaccination was used to elicit a peripheral immune response. Healthy volunteers received a placebo or a vaccination in two separate sessions, after which they completed mood questionnaires and performed an implicit emotional face perception task during functional magnetic resonance imaging (fMRI). The study showed that typhoid vaccination, but not placebo, caused an increase in circulating IL-6 that correlated with mild dysphoria as well as increased activation of the subgenual cingulate cortex in response to faces with negative-valence expressions (e.g., angry or sad), but not neutral or positive expressions (Harrison et al., 2009).

Other studies aimed at understanding molecular mechanisms of inflamed depression have demonstrated that the activation of microglia is associated with changes in monoamine metabolism, said Bullmore. For example, microglia activation is associated with activation of an enzyme called indoleamine 2,3-dioxygenase (IDO), which shunts tryptophan away from serotonin toward the formation of neurotoxic metabolites (Miller and Raison, 2016). This could help explain the relationship between peripheral inflammation and treatment-resistant depression, he said. Following up on that observation, the MRC Consortium has shown that in vitro at least, IDO activation is modulated by anti-inflammatory treatments.

Increased peripheral inflammation may also help explain the links between social and psychological stress and an increased risk of depression, said Bullmore. In one study, chronically stressed teachers were shown to have higher levels of IL-6 than more resilient teachers at baseline, and to react more strongly to the acute stress of a public speaking challenge (Bellingrath et al., 2013).

Clinical experience also suggests that non-psychiatric inflammatory disorders are often associated with depressive symptoms, said Bullmore. In a meta-analysis of anti-inflammatory trials for non-psychiatric conditions, the MRC Consortium demonstrated a reduction in depressive symptoms, although, as Bullmore noted, the trial was not designed to test this effect. He added, however, that the anti-TNFα monoclonal antibody Remicade (infliximab) has well-known but poorly studied effects on mood, producing what clinicians commonly call the "Remicade high." Indeed, a study of TNFα blockade in rheumatoid arthritis patients showed that even before clinical measures of disease activity were affected, subjective ratings of pain were reduced and brain regions involved in pain perception were affected, indicating that TNFα blockade causes functional CNS changes (Hess et al., 2011). Bullmore suggested that future clinical trials of anti-inflammatory drugs for non-psychiatric disorders include brain function and mental-stage changes, in addition to biomarkers of inflammation, to clarify the association between comorbid depression and non-psychiatric disorders.

TNFα blockade as a treatment for major depressive disorder was tested in a phase II clinical trial, but with disappointing results (Raison et al., 2013). However, Bullmore said that in post hoc analysis, a greater improvement in depression scores was observed for individuals with high-baseline CRP, which has led to another study in which participants are stratified according to CRP levels and suboptimal response to standard treatment. While CRP may not be the ideal biomarker, this study demonstrates the potential of biomarkers to improve clinical trials, said Bullmore. The need for better biomarkers prompted the development of BIODEP, a biomarker discovery program funded by the Wellcome Trust Consortium (see Chapter 7), which is looking deep and wide for biomarkers of the peripheral immunophenotype with imaging, cell-based assays, blood- and CSF-based cytokine analyses, and whole blood transcriptomics, and is correlating these measures with clinical and neuropsychological assessments.

Miles Herkenham added that the adaptive immune system has also been shown to affect mood and, in animals, to improve hippocampal neurogenesis, which may be relevant in depression. He suggested that lymphocyte profiling might also represent a useful biomarker. Bullmore said that while the gene expression data suggest that innate immune-related genes from cells of the myeloid lineage were overexpressed more than adaptive immune genes from cells of the lymphoid lineage were underexpressed, current technology lacks the ability to study the adaptive immune system in great detail. The immune system is nothing if not complex and coordinated, he said, so it would be inconceivable that the two parts of the system would not be interacting. However, he said, at this point, pathophysiologically important interactions between the innate and adaptive immune systems are poorly understood.

5

Neuroimaging Biomarkers: Current Initiatives and Opportunities

Highlights

- Nuclear imaging approaches such as positron emission tomography (PET) and single-photon emission computed tomography (SPECT) are potentially capable of monitoring the molecular consequences of neuroinflammation, while magnetic resonance imaging (MRI) enables the visualization of a compromised blood–brain barrier (BBB) (Szardenings).
- MRI combined with iron-oxide labeling allows the visualization of immune cell trafficking, such as microglia accumulation at the site of demyelinated lesions (Absinta, Szardenings).
- TSPO (translocator protein) is a putative biomarker for neuroinflammation, and second-generation PET ligands show an increase in TSPO binding that correlates with symptom severity in Alzheimer's disease (AD), as well as in major depressive episodes (MDEs) (Innis).
- In clinical trials, PET ligands for COX-1 and COX-2, which are components of the cyclooxygenase (COX) system, may be more useful than TSPO as biomarkers of neuroinflammation because they have less variability and more specific cellular localization, and can demonstrate whether a drug is hitting its target (Innis).
- A PET ligand for the purinergic receptor $P2X_7R$, which drives microglia activation, could be useful in the development of therapeutics that target this receptor (Szardenings).
- T2- and T1-weighted MRI with gadolinium infusion are commonly used to diagnose and to monitor multiple sclerosis (MS), but fail to show the overall lesional injury, or chronic inflammation of the MS plaque and within the leptomeninges, which are likely responsible for progressive disease (Absinta, Bar-Or).

- Leptomeningeal inflammation can be imaged using postcontrast 3D T2-FLAIR (fast fluid-attenuated inversion recovery) imaging (Absinta).
- Molecular probes are being developed to enable magnetic resonance imaging of thrombin activity in neuroinflammatory disease (Akassoglou).

NOTE: These points were made by the individual speakers identified above; they are not intended to reflect a consensus among workshop participants.

Many targets and neuroimaging biomarkers of neuroinflammation have been approved for human use, said Anna Katrin Szardenings, director of biomarker operations and imaging at Janssen Research & Development (see Figure 5-1). These include nuclear imaging methods such as PET and SPECT, as well as MRI approaches. Szardenings said both approaches are useful to monitor the pathological consequences of neuroinflammation. Nuclear imaging methods are better equipped to image efflux proteins, while MRI enables the visualization of a compromised BBB and human immune cell trafficking, as well as global atrophy, she said. However, while all of these approaches have proved useful in clinical and research laboratories, particularly in diseases such as MS where there is overt neuroinflammation, Brian Campbell questioned whether they have adequate

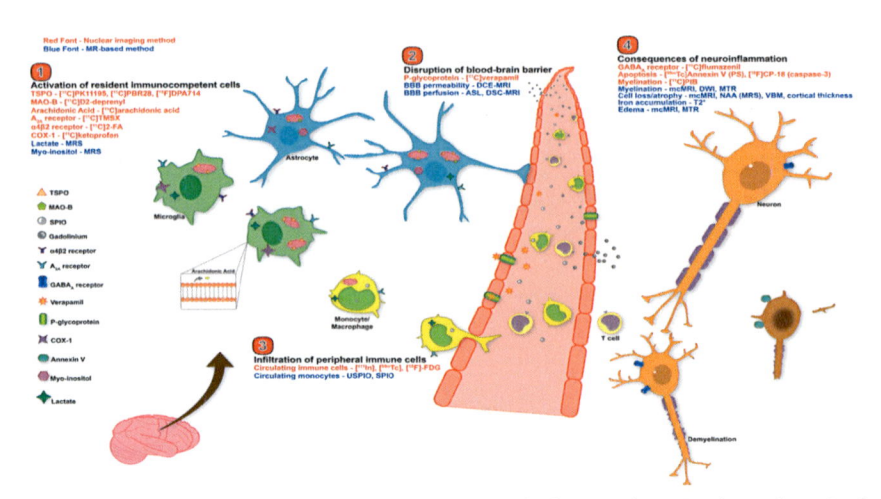

FIGURE 5-1 In vivo imaging of human neuroinflammation. Both nuclear (red font) and magnetic resonance (blue font) imaging methods are used to detect markers of neuroinflammation.
SOURCES: Presentation by Szardenings, March 21, 2017; Albrecht et al., 2016.

sensitivity in diseases where neuroinflammatory changes are more subtle, such as depression, or if these methods are sensitive enough to discriminate subpopulations and their changing microenvironments in diseases such as AD.

NUCLEAR IMAGING APPROACHES

TSPO is a mitochondrial protein that is highly expressed in macrophages, activated microglia, and reactive astrocytes, and thus is a putative biomarker for the activation of the immune system in the brain, said Robert Innis. The first-generation TSPO PET ligand, PK11195, had a low signal-to-noise ratio and gave conflicting results in terms of imaging neuropathology in AD and mild cognitive impairment (MCI). However, Innis said that a second-generation radioligand, PBR28, has a much higher signal-to-noise ratio and shows a significant and widespread increase in TSPO binding in the inferior parietal cortex of patients with AD but not MCI, as well as a correlation with symptom severity (Kreisl et al., 2013). Innis noted that this contrasts with amyloid load as demonstrated with PET imaging, which has never been shown to correlate with cognitive impairment. Moreover, a small longitudinal study in patients with AD and MCI showed that an increase in the amount of TSPO binding correlated with disease progression, suggesting its use as a biomarker of disease progression, said Innis.

Having shown that PBR28 can work as a biomarker in AD, Innis and colleagues investigated its use in MDEs, following up on an earlier study that showed a correlation between TSPO volume and the presence of MDE (Setiawan et al., 2015). Unlike AD, where the neuropathological characteristics have been well defined, MDE has no known neuropathology despite the fact that there is strong evidence that in at least a subset of patients, depression may be linked to peripheral or brain inflammation. The National Institute of Mental Health team demonstrated that unmedicated MDE patients show increased TSPO density compared to healthy controls or patients treated with selective serotonin reuptake inhibitors (SSRIs), suggesting that SSRI treatment itself may influence TSPO density.

Although TSPO may thus be a biomarker of inflammation and might have potential for stratifying patients for clinical trials, Innis said it has limitations because of its high variability. He added that it may not be useful as a tool to demonstrate whether an anti-inflammatory drug is hitting its target because TSPO ligands also act as agonists. However, his team has developed PET ligands for components of the cyclooxygenase system—COX-1 and COX-2—which may be useful in trials of non-steroidal anti-inflammatory drugs because they act as inhibitors of either COX-1 or COX-2. The cyclooxygenase system is responsible for synthesizing inflammatory mediators called prostanoids from arachidonic acid, said Innis. COX-1 and COX-2 are present in different cell types and have different functions. Innis believes that because of its cellular localization, COX-1 may be more useful as a biomarker in neuroinflammatory disorders. Uptake of COX-1 radioligands is specific and is blocked even by low doses of highly selective COX-1 antagonists. Innis and colleagues will soon be starting first-in-human studies of these various radioligands.

Szardenings, along with Hartmuth Kolb and colleagues at Janssen Neuroscience and the University of Leuven, have focused efforts on developing the purinergic receptor $P2X_7R$ as a PET tracer to be used in conjunction with the development of a therapeutic compound. In rat models, $P2X_7R$ is expressed at low levels throughout the brain, primarily in microglia and astrocytes (Choi et al., 2007). According to Szardenings, $P2X_7R$ expression drives microglia activation, activating the inflammasome and interleukin (IL)-1β secretion, thus making it a relevant target for monitoring neuroinflammation. Preclinical studies indicate that the ligand in development, known as 739, hits the target with minimal non-specific binding and can be blocked with an antagonist, she said. Following primate studies that demonstrated dose-dependent target occupancy, the team tested the ligand in an inflammatory rat model, where they showed that inducing neuroinflammation by injecting lipopolysaccharide locally into the striatum was associated with an increased uptake of 739, and that the antagonist blocked this effect, indicating that 739 may be useful to measure target engagement of $P2X_7R$ therapeutics and to image neuroinflammation. However, Szardenings noted that because $P2X_7R$ is evenly distributed throughout the brain, there is no reference region to allow calculation of occupancy and aid in image analysis. Future efforts will compare PET images using 739 to other markers of inflammation, said Szardenings.

MAGNETIC RESONANCE IMAGING APPROACHES

As mentioned in Chapter 4, MRI has become the predominant tool for diagnosing MS. Indeed, said Amit Bar-Or, axial brain MRI in patients with MS shows bright hyperintensity on T2-weighted images, demonstrating over time that the disease is dynamic, multifocal, and diffuse. Moreover, gadolinium enhancement demonstrates a breach of the integrity of the BBB, which is thought to reflect perivascular inflammation; MRI also is used to assess brain atrophy as a measure of global injury, although this measure is affected by an individual's level of hydration, he said. In addition, Bar-Or said that standard MRI sequences fail to show a substantial degree of injury that is interlesional.

Martina Absinta of the Translational Neuroradiology Section at the National Institute of Neurological Disorders and Stroke showed time-lapse MRI from more than 100 gadolinium-enhanced scans from MS patients collected over 24 years. These scans demonstrate the highly inflammatory nature of MS, the progressive enlargement of the ventricles suggesting ongoing atrophy over time, and neurodegeneration. However, in addition to the acute inflammation seen in these images, which is associated with the opening of the BBB, Absinta said that chronic inflammation occurs behind a partially intact BBB at the plaque level and within the leptomeninges. This chronic inflammation is invisible to gadolinium-based MRI, although it is likely responsible for progressive disease.

Pathological studies show that chronic, active demyelinated lesions can be further visualized using iron staining to show the accumulation of activated microglia at their edges, said Absinta. She noted that chronic inactive lesions, in contrast, are still completely demyelinated, but are devoid of inflammatory cells. To see this pathology in living patients, she and her colleagues are using 7-Tesla susceptibility-based MRI, which is sensitive to paramagnetic substances such as iron (Absinta et al., 2013). These images show a dark rim around the lesion indicative of microglial accumulation. In a longitudinal study of newly formed lesions imaged over 18 months, this imaging modality allowed them to identify three different scenarios of lesion evolution as well as the propensity to repair. Then, using postmortem MRI, they confirmed that the worst of these lesions, where the dark rim persists, are completely demyelinated and surrounded by activated microglia (Absinta et al., 2016). They concluded that chronic inflammation develops within the first 3 months of lesion onset and marks the failure of early lesion repair.

In another series of studies, Absinta and colleagues are using MR techniques to image chronic inflammation within the leptomeningeal compartment because pathology studies have shown that meningeal inflammation is a key and persistent driver of MS pathogenesis both early in the disease and at later progressive stages. The technique they use is called postcontrast 3D T2-FLAIR (fast fluid-attenuated inversion recovery). In a study of 299 MS patients, they demonstrated that focal areas of perivascular leptomeningeal enhancement are much more prevalent in the progressive phase of disease, and that patients with leptomeningeal enhancement were more disabled, older, had long disease duration, and had lower brain and cortical volumes (Absinta et al., 2015). Two autopsy cases, in combination with the in vivo data, confirmed the role of leptomeningeal enhancement as a biomarker for meningeal inflammation associated with the opening of the BBB, said Absinta. She added that other chronic neuroinflammatory conditions show a similar pattern of blood–meningeal barrier impairment due to meningeal inflammation using this technique, suggesting that it may be useful for patient selection and stratification in clinical trials of disease-modifying treatments for chronic inflammation. Correlating this imaging biomarker with cytokine profiles in the cerebrospinal fluid might also lead to a better understanding of what drives cortical demyelination in MS, she said.

Katerina Akassoglou and colleagues, in collaboration with Roger Tsien and Michael Whitney at the University of California, San Diego, also developed molecular probes that may be used with MRI to monitor thrombin activity in neuroinflammatory disease. As described in Chapter 3, soluble fibrinogen acts with thrombin to form insoluble fibrin, which plays a role in blood clotting and is highly proinflammatory, said Akassoglou. In the experimental autoimmune encephalomyelitis mouse model of MS, the thrombin probe they developed accumulates at the site of demyelinating lesions and correlates with demyelination as well as activation of innate immunity and neurodegeneration (Davalos et al., 2014) (see Figure 5-2). The technology is currently being tested in clinical applications in cancer, and could provide a sensitive tool to be able to detect early changes in clotting and fibrin deposition that could indicate very early BBB leakage in the course of MS, said Akassoglou.

The importance of fibrin deposition during the course of MS is also substantiated by proteomic analysis in human MS lesions, which demonstrate excessive and persistent fibrin deposition in pre-active, active, chronic, and chronic inactive MS lesions (Claudio et al., 1989; Han et al., 2008; Kirk et al., 2003; Marik et al., 2007; Vos et al., 2005). Akassoglou added that numerous neuropathological studies also show the presence of fibrin in AD (Cortes-Canteli, 2015; Lee at al., 2007; Ryu et al., 2009),

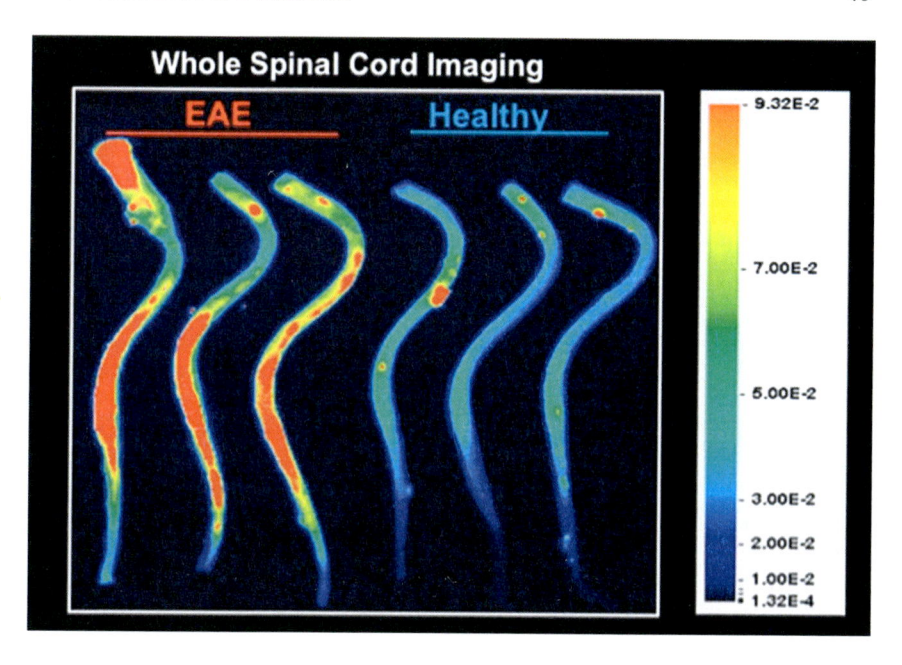

FIGURE 5-2 Coagulation activity in the central nervous system as a sensitive imaging biomarker. Whole spinal cord scans from experimental autoimmune encephalomyelitis (EAE) mice and healthy controls injected with a fluorescently labeled thrombin probe demonstrate the potential to use this probe to detect early changes in clotting and fibrin deposition indicative of blood–brain barrier leakage.
SOURCE: Presentation by Akassoglou, March 21, 2017.

which correlates with microglia activation and dystrophy, a sign of microglial senescence in the aging brain (Streit et al., 2004). Fibrin and activation of coagulation could be a common thread and therapeutic target among neurological diseases with vascular alterations, she concluded.

6

Cerebrospinal Fluid and Other Fluid Biomarkers: Current Initiatives and Opportunities

Highlights

- An Alzheimer's disease (AD) biomarker discovery program identified a panel of plasma and cerebrospinal fluid (CSF) proteins that serve as predictive biomarkers in AD (Perrin).
- Because of small sample sizes, insufficient validation of assays, and lack of standardization, there remains no consensus in the literature regarding CSF and plasma biomarkers of neuroinflammation (Campbell).
- Two consortia have been established to identify panels of neuroinflammatory biomarkers for neurodegenerative diseases and mood disorders (Bullmore, Campbell).
- Secreted biomarkers of neuron–microglia interactions are being explored as a way to track neuroinflammation in schizophrenia and other central nervous system (CNS) diseases (McCarroll).
- The gene for a component of the complement cascade, which has been implicated in synapse pruning, appears to have the strongest genetic influence (among common variants, at a population level) on the development of schizophrenia (McCarroll).
- A novel technology called Drop-seq enables high-throughput, single-cell analyses of gene expression; the technology is being further extended to the analysis of archival (fresh-frozen) brain samples and may enable the identification and interpretation of new biomarkers (McCarroll).

NOTE: These points were made by the individual speakers identified above; they are not intended to reflect a consensus among workshop participants.

In CNS disorders that have a neuroinflammatory or immune component, quantification of analytes in the CSF and blood may enable assessment of the peripheral versus central immune response, determine whether these analytes correlate with development or progression of disease, and help show if inflammation in the peripheral compartment reflects what is going on in the brain, said Brian Campbell. Indeed, some of the strongest evidence supporting the role of neuroinflammation in CNS disease has arisen from biomarker discovery programs. For example, Richard Perrin described an AD biomarker discovery program he conducted with colleagues at the Knight Alzheimer's Disease Research Center at Washington University (Craig-Schapiro et al., 2011). Using a multiplex immunoassay (Luminex) platform applied to 333 paired CSF and plasma samples from cognitively normal to mildly demented individuals, the researchers measured 190 analytes thought to be important in the disease. These analytes included cytokines, chemokines, metabolic markers, growth factors, and other proteins. The studies indicated that a panel of plasma or CSF proteins can be used to predict who has existing brain amyloid or will likely become amyloid positive and who will likely develop dementia (see Figure 6-1). Markers that predicted conversion to amyloid positivity included anti-inflammatory markers in the CSF and both pro- and anti-inflammatory markers in the plasma, indicating that peripheral inflammation is an early event in AD pathogenesis. Once people develop amyloid plaques, anti-inflammatory markers are seen in both the CSF and plasma along with markers of low adiposity and low insulin signaling. Among those who are likely to develop dementia in the next 3 to 4 years, Perrin said there is a robust neuroinflammatory signal, especially in the CSF, as well as evidence of vasculopathy that may be related to blood–brain barrier (BBB) breakdown and hypothalamic, pituitary, and metabolic changes. Perrin maintained that the variability in levels of inflammatory biomarkers over the course of disease argues against the disease being a continual process, as has been proposed.

However, Campbell said there remains a lack of consensus in the literature about most CSF and plasma markers that have been measured thus far, which stems largely from small sample sizes, insufficient validation of assays, and lack of standardization in terms of analytes measured and collection, handling, and storage of samples. The Alzheimer's Disease Neuroimaging Initiative (ADNI), a public–private partnership established by the NIA and the Foundation for the National Institutes of Health (FNIH) in 2004, specifically addressed these issues of standardization

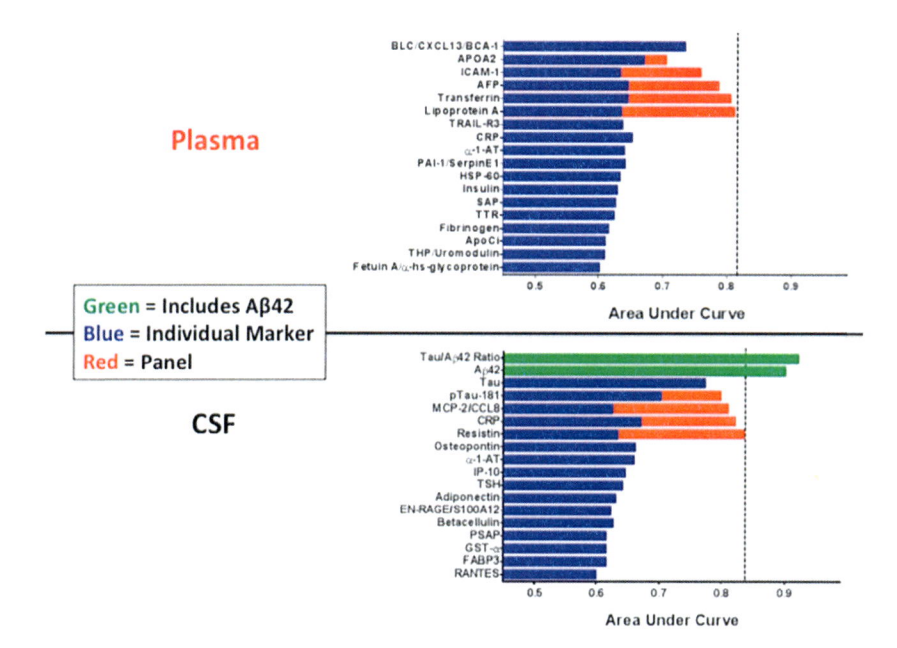

FIGURE 6-1 Predicting amyloid status using panels of plasma (upper graph) and cerebrospinal fluid (CSF) (lower graph) biomarkers. Blue bars show the prediction level (area under the curve or AUC) of individual novel markers. Green bars in lower graph show the AUC of the "gold standard" predictors, tau/Aβ_{42} or Aβ_{42} alone. Red bars show the stepwise construction of the panel, demonstrating that even without Aβ_{42}, panels of CSF and plasma biomarkers provide good predictors of amyloid status.
SOURCE: Presentation by Perrin, March 21, 2017.

and validation of AD biomarkers, noted Eliezer Masliah, director of the Division of Neuroscience at NIA. More recently, other consortia have also emerged to build on ADNI's efforts to standardize and validate assays.

Campbell and Edward Bullmore described two other consortia established over the past 5 years specifically to identify inflammatory biomarkers for CNS diseases: the Wellcome Trust Consortium for Neuroimmunology of Mood Disorders and Alzheimer's Disease, and the FNIH Biomarkers Consortium's project on Inflammatory Markers for Early Detection and Subtyping of Neurodegenerative and Mood Disorders. The operations of these two consortia are discussed in more detail in Chapter 7. In both programs, rather than taking the relatively agnostic approach of measuring a large number of analytes across different categories as was previously described by Perrin, they have focused specifically on a select group of analytes related to inflammation. Perrin said these are complimentary approaches.

The FNIH Biomarkers Consortium project selected inflammatory analytes, such as cytokines and chemokines (C-reactive protein, interleukin [IL]-1β, IL-6, TNFα, IL-10, sIL-6R, and IL-1RA), that will be assessed using enzyme-linked immunosorbent assay (ELISA)-based technologies, as well as tryptophan and kynurenine metabolites, which are effector molecules for the immune system that will be assessed using mass spectrometry assays, said Campbell. He said the Consortium hopes to identify a panel of inflammatory biomarkers—a biosignature—that has sufficient power to be used at the individual patient level for diagnosis, subtyping, and monitoring disease progression or response to therapy. Prior results in bipolar disorder studies support this approach, said Campbell (Brietzke et al., 2012; McIntyre et al., 2014). The Wellcome Trust has selected an overlapping set of inflammatory biomarkers to assess. For major depressive disorder, these include CRP, IL-1β, IL-6, TNF-α, IL-10, and tryptophan and kynurenine metabolites, he said.

Proteomic analysis also suggests that fibrinogen, fibrin degradation products, or other products of the coagulation cascade may also be useful as plasma biomarkers in multiple sclerosis and AD (Han et al., 2008; Lee et al., 2007), said Katerina Akassoglou; however, these are not currently included in either of the programs mentioned above.

NOVEL APPROACHES TO IDENTIFYING GENETIC AND MOLECULAR MARKERS OF NEUROINFLAMMATION

Steve McCarroll is pursuing a different approach to identify genetic and molecular markers of neuroinflammation in schizophrenia and other CNS diseases by assessing secreted biomarkers of neuron–microglia interactions. Schizophrenia is a heritable but extremely polygenic illness shaped by genetic variation in at least 100 loci, said McCarroll. The strongest genetic influence appears to come from genes involved in immunity and infection that reside within the major histocompatibility complex locus on chromosome 6, in particular, the complement component 4 (C4) gene, which has been implicated in the pruning of synapses. McCarroll and colleagues have shown that this gene has many structurally different allelic forms that result in different levels of C4A and C4B expression, and that schizophrenia is associated with particular variants that lead to elevated C4A expression (Sekar et al., 2016). More recent work from the lab of McCarroll's colleague Michael Carroll has shown that microglia engulf synapses decorated with C4A.

These discoveries, combined with the knowledge that in humans, key cortical regions undergo maturation and pruning during adolescence and early adulthood, which is also when schizophrenia typically presents, suggest that schizophrenia may result or worsen when a normal developmental process is recruited into pathophysiology. Because C4 is a secreted molecule, it also suggested that it might be possible to "listen in" on the conversation between neurons and microglia by assessing C4 levels in the CSF, said McCarroll. Indeed, their recent paper (Sekar et al., 2016) showed that in postmortem brain tissue, C4A RNA expression is about 40 percent higher in patients with schizophrenia than in normal controls. McCarroll added that this effect is much stronger than the 20 percent effect predicted by the genetic relationship to C4 (i.e., the fact that schizophrenia patients on average have high-C4A-expressing alleles). Because there are limits to the value of a measurement in postmortem brain tissue, McCarroll's lab has been measuring C4 and other potentially relevant analytes in CSF. They have shown that when postmortem tissue and CSF are both available from the same individuals, the protein levels in CSF correlate strongly with levels of RNA in cortical tissue. Because the cortex is the largest source of CSF C4, this suggests that CSF may provide information about C4 expression in brain tissue. Moreover, unlike C4 alleles, C4 protein levels in CSF are a potential biomarker for dynamic processes that are shaped by genes, environment, and development. Plasma levels of C4, however, are unlikely to be informative because C4 does not routinely cross the BBB, said McCarroll.

McCarroll and colleagues have recently initiated an analysis of C4 as well as other proteins and small-molecule metabolites in a set of CSF samples from youths with attenuated psychotic symptoms who are at ultra-high risk for progression to frank psychosis and schizophrenia. They also hope to apply this approach to a large number of samples from healthy individuals to map out the natural history of these analytes and establish normative values.

McCarroll's lab has also developed a novel technology to enable high-throughput, single-cell analyses of gene expression to study circuitry change during critical periods of development. This technology, called "Drop-seq," isolates individual cells in millions of tiny droplets, uses beads to deliver different molecular barcodes to each droplet, and then analyzes the messenger RNA (mRNA) transcripts from thousands of cells simultaneously while remembering the source of each transcript because of the bar code (Macosko et al., 2015). They then use machine-learning approaches to classify cells into groups or types based on their genome-wide transcriptional patterns, allowing them to create atlases of cell types and cell-type-specific gene expression in different tissues. McCarroll's lab has been using Drop-seq to identify biomarkers of developmental critical periods—the time in development when the synaptic circuitry is changing very quickly—in both neurons and glia. Because many of these mRNAs encode secreted proteins that can be detected in CSF, McCarroll believes the Drop-seq data nominate new CSF biomarkers and aid in the interpretation of CSF biomarker data, making it possible to identify which cells are the source of a particular biomarker and what distinguishes cells that express that biomarker from cells that do not.

7

Potential Mechanisms for Moving Forward

Highlights

- The search for biomarkers of neuroinflammation encompasses two objectives that may or may not be achievable in parallel: (1) elucidating pathophysiological mechanisms and (2) predicting a treatment response (Bar-Or, Bullmore, Campbell, Perrin, Samad).
- Biomarkers are needed to stratify patients into subpopulations for clinical trials, yet there is little agreement on the best strategy to identify these biomarkers (Hyman, Miller, Potter).
- For neuropsychiatric diseases such as depression, there may already be biomarkers of neuroinflammation that can be used for subtyping, even as research continues on the underlying mechanisms (Miller).
- Some consortia have already been established to identify biomarkers of neuroinflammation, but others may be needed to address the challenges mentioned above, as well as to devise strategies to deal with increasing amounts of data (Bullmore, Campbell, Hyman, Samad, Stevens).
- A new consortium that would conduct transcriptomic studies on cells and cerebrospinal fluid (CSF) from normal individuals as well as those with selected diseases, sharing cells, CSF, and data about candidate biomarkers, would be beneficial to the field (Hyman, Potter).

NOTE: These points were made by the individual speakers identified above; they are not intended to reflect a consensus among workshop participants.

Brian Campbell commented that the search for biomarkers encompasses two different objectives: (1) to understand more about the pathophysiology of disease process and (2) to find biomarkers that could be useful in terms of predicting treatment response. These two objectives may merit different strategies, he said. Edward Bullmore suggested that this challenge will be easier to manage for therapeutically focused biomarkers by selecting a particular molecule and then identifying a few biomarkers relevant to the target. Amit Bar-Or noted that although the therapeutic context may provide a more focused opportunity to look at a target or pathway, it could still fall short of elucidating the relevant biological pathways. He argued that a more comprehensive model will be needed to capture the cellular responses and related molecules that comprise pathways. Richard Perrin added that more foundational work is also needed before the neuroinflammatory markers can be used intelligently in clinical trials, adding that he believes the field is close to achieving an adequate understanding of neuroinflammation to move forward.

Tarek Samad said that in order to meet the above objectives, other challenges will need to be addressed: selecting appropriate disease subpopulations, determining the stage or stages of disease to investigate, selecting appropriate measuring tools, and defining a positive outcome with regard to measuring brain neuroimmune tone. While these gaps suggest a development pathway that focuses on disease biology, Samad said that in order to gain enthusiasm and traction from the pharmaceutical industry, a well defined clinical path forward will be required. Bar-Or suggested that there may be a way to combine the broad strategy that Samad mentioned with a shorter-term strategy that could provide incentives for industry. This should include concerted efforts to (1) look at markers in both the periphery and the central nervous system (CNS), he said, including soluble phase markers in both the CSF and blood, as well as cell-based markers, and (2) examine both disease-related and treatment-related differences.

William Potter reiterated what several speakers mentioned throughout the day, that one of the biggest areas of need is biomarkers that can stratify subtypes of patients in treatment for psychiatric or neurological disorders. However, he said there is less agreement on the best way to identify these biomarkers. One option would be to predefine a set of potential analytes and use multiplex technologies, such as expression profiling, proteomics, or other omics approaches, to build composite measures that would allow stratification of individuals. Alternatively, a more hypothesis-driven approach could be used to develop a better understanding of the function of different cell types in the brain. Both approaches may be valuable, and some large tissue repositories are available to conduct these studies. However, given the limited resources available, it may be necessary to choose one over another, said Potter. Andrew Miller argued that both approaches are necessary because picking a set of biomarkers now based on the limited data available could be dangerous. He advocated for more hypothesis testing with a discovery-based analytic strategy. Hyman said the correct approach may differ depending on the disease.

In terms of differences between therapeutic and scientific biomarkers, Miller also challenged workshop participants to think differently about functional disorders that fall into the realm of psychiatry and formal neurological disorders where there is clear pathology in the brain. For neuropsychiatric disorders, such as depression, there may be relatively simple solutions available today to identify inflammation, and these may be proxies for what is going on in the brain. For example, it is now widely accepted that a systemic biomarker of neuroinflammation, C-reactive protein, can be used to predict response to selective serotonin reuptake inhibitors, so subgrouping patients and assessing their responses to different treatment paradigms could accelerate treatment development, even as research continues to try to understand the cell-mediated immune processes that also contribute to neuroinflammation, he said.

Another major concern raised by Samad is how to manage the data already collected, including data that already exist within pharmaceutical companies. Hyman agreed, noting that underlying all of the challenges mentioned the need to better understand human biology. The appropriate specimens are precious and rare, he said, thus demanding a consortial process that can centralize the data production and analysis. Such a process was used successfully in the Alzheimer's Disease Neuroimaging Initiative (ADNI), for example, when investigators from multiple stakeholder groups and disciplines got together and laid out very clear questions, said Potter. This allowed the ADNI investigators to decide whether or not the measures were informative enough to answer those questions. While laying out the questions may be possible in the area of neuroinflammation, Potter wondered whether the techniques currently available to study brain microglia and astrocytes are adequate.

Beth Stevens suggested that these problems can all be addressed by bringing together the right consortia or group of people to do this work collaboratively by coming at problems from different perspectives and with different types of expertise. In addition, Bar-Or challenged the attendees to think about ways of bringing together and mandating certain kinds of cohesion so that the same question can be asked identically across different samples collected from different diseases.

CONSORTIAL EFFORTS TO IDENTIFY AND VALIDATE BIOMARKERS OF NEUROINFLAMMATION

Campbell advocated for the use of precompetitive, public–private consortia to facilitate the development of inflammation biomarkers, noting that multiple organizations with areas of common interest may be able to pool the necessary resources for well-powered studies that most likely will incur enormous costs and take years to complete. Such consortia will bring value to the entire field by promoting greater visibility, increasing the power of studies by enabling the enrollment of large numbers of participants, aggregating financial resources as well as the human resources of people with different skill sets, and reducing the risk of investment for individual partners, said Campbell. Eliezer Masliah noted that for several years the National Institute on Aging has been funding studies on CSF and fluid biomarkers conducted by public–private consortia.

Within the area of neuroinflammation, two consortia that have been established in recent years were discussed in Chapter 6. Campbell described one of these, the Foundation for the National Institutes of Health (FNIH) Biomarkers Consortium's project, which will focus on blood and CSF biomarkers (thus, both peripheral and central immune responses) in Alzheimer's disease (AD) and major depressive disorder (MDD). This project was established to develop biosignatures of neuroinflammation in CNS disorders, ultimately narrowing down their scope to one neurodegenerative disease, AD, and one psychiatric disorder, MDD, said Campbell. He described the two different enzyme-linked immunosorbent assay platforms and a mass spectrometry platform that will be used to measure the selected neuroinflammatory cytokines and chemokines. He also outlined their three aims: (1) to validate the selected assay platforms with respect to sensitivity, linear range, reproducibility, and other parameters; (2) to develop inflammatory biosignatures based on a training set of samples; and (3) to confirm these biosignatures in a validation cohort of patients.

The other is the Wellcome Trust Consortium for Neuroimmunology of Mood Disorders and Alzheimer's Disease. Bullmore said that in 2014 the Medical Research Council in the United Kingdom agreed to fund this consortium to focus on immunologic approaches to treat neuropsychiatric disorders, bringing together several academic centers in the United Kingdom with two pharmaceutical partners, GlaxoSmithKline and Janssen. The goal of this consortium was to build confidence in the concept of using immunotherapeutics in psychiatry by reanalyzing existing data from clinical trials and microarray datasets, as well as by conducting some novel experimental work, said Bullmore. He described the overall program, which includes the preclinical testing of new molecules contributed by the pharma partners as well as biomarker discovery in clinical studies aimed at exploring whether biomarkers can demonstrate a relationship between peripheral and central inflammation as well as a possible relationship between therapeutic resistance to antidepressants and peripheral inflammation. Ultimately, he said the consortium hopes to take one of the new molecules tested preclinically into an experimental medicine or proof-of-concept study for treatment-resistant depression. He added that in 2015 the consortium was expanded to include a wider range of activities in mood disorders and AD with funding from the Wellcome Trust and the addition of two more pharmaceutical partners, Lundbeck and Pfizer.

Campbell highlighted the opportunities for synergy between the efforts of the FNIH Biomarkers Consortium and the Wellcome Trust Initiative (see Figure 7-1). He said, for example, that it may be possible to include samples from the Wellcome Trust in the Biomarkers Consortium's assay evaluation to provide a stronger synergized dataset. The Wellcome Trust has selected an overlapping set of fluid-based inflammatory biomarkers to assess in MDD patients. They are also including TSPO (translocator protein) imaging as an inflammation biomarker, whereas the FNIH Biomarkers Consortium has prioritized its work to the assessment of fluid biomarkers. Campbell said that cell-based measurements in the periphery and CSF could be incorporated in the future if the scientific evidence points in that direction and if additional funds are procured.

Beyond these existing consortia, Hyman proposed another large consortium to conduct transcriptomic studies in normal individuals as well as those with selected diseases, looking at cells and CSF, and sharing data about candidate biomarkers. Potter agreed, noting that it would be necessary to determine what questions to ask that would be informative, and whether adequate techniques are available to address those questions.

Comparison between Wellcome Trust Biomarkers Consortium and FNIH Biomarkers Consortium
- Both efforts evaluate plasma and CSF samples from major depressive disorder (MDD) patients
- Overlap in some MDD inflammation biomarker panel endpoints (in red)
- MSD platform will be evaluated in both consortia

Key differences
- Technical validation of assay platforms
- Evaluation of SiMoA platform performance included in FNIH Biomarkers
- Evaluation and comparison of Alzheimer's Disease (AD) plasma and CSF samples

Inflammation Biomarkers

	FNIH Biomarkers	Wellcome Trust
AD	CRP, TNF-α, IL-1b, IL-6, IL-10, sIL-6R, IL-1RA, CD40 KP metabolites	TSPO imaging
MDD	CRP, TNF-α, IL-1b, IL-6, IL-10, sIL-6R, IL-1RA, CD40 KP metabolites	CRP, IFN-g, TNF-α, IL-1β, IL-6, IL-10 KP metabolites TSPO imaging

Opportunity to capitalize on synergies
- Opportunity exists to include biosamples from Wellcome Trust consortium in FNIH Biomarkers Consortium assays to compare outcomes

FIGURE 7-1 Synergizing the efforts of two consortia developing plasma and cerebrospinal fluid (CSF) biomarkers of neuroinflammation. Key commonalities and differences between the Foundation for the National Institutes of Health (FNIH) Biomarkers Consortium and the Wellcome Trust initiative are outlined at the top of the figure. As summarized in the table, both consortia have separate but complementary projects to develop plasma and CSF biomarkers of neuroinflammation in Alzheimer's disease (AD) and major depressive disorder (MDD), offering opportunities for synergy by sharing data and samples.
SOURCE: Presentation by Campbell, March 21, 2017.

A
References

Absinta, M., P. Sati, M. I. Gaitan, P. Maggi, I. C. Cortese, M. Filippi, and D. S. Reich. 2013. Seven-Tesla phase imaging of acute multiple sclerosis lesions: A new window into the inflammatory process. *Annals of Neurology* 74(5):669-678.

Absinta, M., L. Vuolo, A. Rao, G. Nair, P. Sati, I. C. Cortese, J. Ohayon, K. Fenton, M. I. Reyes-Mantilla, D. Maric, P. A. Calabresi, J. A. Butman, C. A. Pardo, and D. S. Reich. 2015. Gadolinium-based MRI characterization of leptomeningeal inflammation in multiple sclerosis. *Neurology* 85(1):18-28.

Absinta, M., P. Sati, M. Schindler, E. C. Leibovitch, J. Ohayon, T. Wu, A. Meani, M. Filippi, S. Jacobson, I. C. Cortese, and D. S. Reich. 2016. Persistent 7-Tesla phase rim predicts poor outcome in new multiple sclerosis patient lesions. *Journal of Clinical Investigation* 126(7):2597-2609.

Adams, R. A., J. Bauer, M. J. Flick, S. L. Sikorski, T. Nuriel, H. Lassmann, J. L. Degen, and K. Akassoglou. 2007. The fibrin-derived gamma377-395 peptide inhibits microglia activation and suppresses relapsing paralysis in central nervous system autoimmune disease. *Journal of Experimental Medicine* 204(3):571-582.

Albrecht, D. S., C. Granziera, J. M. Hooker, and M. L. Loggia. 2016. In vivo imaging of human neuroinflammation. *ACS Chemical Neuroscience* 7(4):470-483.

Atkins, H. L., M. Bowman, D. Allan, G. Anstee, D. L. Arnold, A. Bar-Or, I. Bence-Bruckler, P. Birch, C. Bredeson, J. Chen, D. Fergusson, M. Halpenny, L. Hamelin, L. Huebsch, B. Hutton, P. Laneuville, Y. Lapierre, H. Lee, L. Martin, S. McDiarmid, P. O'Connor, T. Ramsay, M. Sabloff, L. Walker, and M. S. Freedman. 2016. Immunoablation and autologous haemopoietic stem-cell transplantation for aggressive multiple sclerosis: A multicentre single-group Phase 2 trial. *The Lancet* 388(10044):576-585.

Bar-Or, A., L. Fawaz, B. Fan, P. J. Darlington, A. Rieger, C. Ghorayeb, P. A. Calabresi, E. Waubant, S. L. Hauser, J. Zhang, and C. H. Smith. 2010. Abnormal B-cell cytokine responses a trigger of T-cell-mediated disease in MS? *Annals of Neurology* 67(4):452-461.

Bellingrath, S., N. Rohleder, and B. M. Kudielka. 2013. Effort-reward-imbalance in healthy teachers is associated with higher LPS-stimulated production and lower glucocorticoid sensitivity of interleukin-6 in vitro. *Biological Psychology* 92(2):403-409.

Bianchin, M. M., H. M. Capella, D. L. Chaves, M. Steindel, E. C. Grisard, G. G. Ganev, J. P. da Silva, Jr., S. Neto Evaldo, M. A. Poffo, R. Walz, C. G. Carlotti, Jr., and A. C. Sakamoto. 2004. Nasu-Hakola disease (polycystic lipomembranous osteodysplasia with sclerosing leukoencephalopathy—PLOSL): A dementia associated with bone cystic lesions. From clinical to genetic and molecular aspects. *Cellular and Molecular Neurobiology* 24(1):1-24.

Brietzke, E., R. B. Mansur, J. K. Soczynska, F. Kapczinski, R. A. Bressan, and R. S. McIntyre. 2012. Towards a multifactorial approach for prediction of bipolar disorder in at risk populations. *Journal of Affective Disorders* 140(1):82-91.

Bullmore, E. T., and M. E. Lynall. 2014. Immunologic therapeutics and psychotic disorders. *Biological Psychiatry* 75(4):260-261.

Choi, H. B., J. K. Ryu, S. U. Kim, and J. G. McLarnon. 2007. Modulation of the purinergic p2x7 receptor attenuates lipopolysaccharide-mediated microglial activation and neuronal damage in inflamed brain. *Journal of Neuroscience* 27(18):4957-4968.

Ciccarelli, O., F. Barkhof, B. Bodini, N. De Stefano, X. Golay, K. Nicolay, D. Pelletier, P. J. Pouwels, S. A. Smith, C. A. Wheeler-Kingshott, B. Stankoff, T. Yousry, and D. H. Miller. 2014. Pathogenesis of multiple sclerosis: Insights from molecular and metabolic imaging. *Lancet Neurology* 13(8):807-822.

Claudio, L., Y. Kress, W. T. Norton, and C. F. 1989. Brosnan. Increased vesicular transport and decreased mitochondrial content in blood-brain barrier endothelial cells during experimental autoimmune encephalomyelitis. *American Journal of Pathology* 135(6):1157-1168.

Cortes-Canteli, M., J. Paul, E. H. Norris, R. Bronstein, H. J. Ahn, D. Zamolodchikov, S. Bhuvanendran, K. M. Fenz, and S. Strickland. 2010. Fibrinogen and beta-amyloid association alters thrombosis and fibrinolysis: A possible contributing factor to Alzheimer's disease. *Neuron* 66(5):695-709.

Cortes-Canteli, M., L. Mattei, A. T. Richards, E. H. Norris, and S. Strickland. 2015. Fibrin deposited in the Alzheimer's disease brain promotes neuronal degeneration. *Neurobiology of Aging* 36(2):608-617.

Craig-Schapiro, R., M. Kuhn, C. Xiong, E. H. Pickering, J. Liu, T. P. Misko, R. J. Perrin, K. R. Bales, H. Soares, A. M. Fagan, and D. M. Holtzman. 2011. Multiplexed immunoassay panel identifies novel CSF biomarkers for Alzheimer's disease diagnosis and prognosis. *PLoS ONE* 6(4):e18850.

Daneman, R., L. Zhou, A. A. Kebede, and B. A. Barres. 2010. Pericytes are required for blood–brain barrier integrity during embryogenesis. *Nature* 468(7323):562-566.

Davalos, D., J. K. Ryu, M. Merlini, K. M. Baeten, N. Le Moan, M. A. Petersen, T. J. Deerinck, D. S. Smirnoff, C. Bedard, H. Hakozaki, S. Gonias Murray, J. B. Ling, H. Lassmann, J. L. Degen, M. H. Ellisman, and K. Akassoglou. 2012. Fibrinogen-induced perivascular microglial clustering is required for the development of axonal damage in neuroinflammation. *Nature Communications* 3:1227.

Davalos, D., K. M. Baeten, M. A. Whitney, E. S. Mullins, B. Friedman, E. S. Olson, J. K. Ryu, D. S. Smirnoff, M. A. Petersen, C. Bedard, J. L. Degen, R. Y. Tsien, and K. Akassoglou. 2014. Early detection of thrombin activity in neuroinflammatory disease. *Annals of Neurology* 75(2):303-308.

Fagan, A. M., and R. J. Perrin. 2012. Upcoming candidate cerebrospinal fluid biomarkers of Alzheimer's disease. *Biomarkers in Medicine* 6(4):455-476.

Ferguson, S., B. Mouzon, D. Paris, D. Aponte, L. Abdullah, W. Stewart, M. Mullan, and F. Crawford. 2017. Acute or delayed treatment with anatabine improves spatial memory and reduces pathological sequelae at late timepoints after repetitive mild traumatic brain injury. *Journal of Neurotrauma* 34(8):1676-1691.

Guerreiro, R., A. Wojtas, J. Bras, M. Carrasquillo, E. Rogaeva, E. Majounie, C. Cruchaga, C. Sassi, J. S. Kauwe, S. Younkin, L. Hazrati, J. Collinge, J. Pocock, T. Lashley, J. Williams, J. C. Lambert, P. Amouyel, A. Goate, R. Rademakers, K. Morgan, J. Powell, P. St. George-Hyslop, A. Singleton, J. Hardy, and Alzheimer Genetic Analysis Group. 2013. TREM2 variants in Alzheimer's disease. *New England Journal of Medicine* 368(2):117-127.

Haapakoski, R., J. Mathieu, K. P. Ebmeier, H. Alenius, and M. Kivimaki. 2015. Cumulative meta-analysis of interleukins 6 and 1beta, tumour necrosis factor alpha and C-reactive protein in patients with major depressive disorder. *Brain Behavior and Immunity* 49:206-215.

Han, M. H., S. I. Hwang, D. B. Roy, D. H. Lundgren, J. V. Price, S. S. Ousman, G. H. Fernald, B. Gerlitz, W. H. Robinson, S. E. Baranzini, B. W. Grinnell, C. S. Raine, R. A. Sobel, D. K. Han, and L. Steinman. 2008. Proteomic analysis of active multiple sclerosis lesions reveals therapeutic targets. *Nature* 451(7182):1076-1081.

Harrison, N. A., L. Brydon, C. Walker, M. A. Gray, A. Steptoe, and H. D. Critchley. 2009. Inflammation causes mood changes through alterations in subgenual cingulate activity and mesolimbic connectivity. *Biological Psychiatry* 66(5):407-414.

Hauser, S. L., A. Bar-Or, G. Comi, G. Giovannoni, H. P. Hartung, B. Hemmer, F. Lublin, X. Montalban, K. W. Rammohan, K. Selmaj, A. Traboulsee, J. S. Wolinsky, D. L. Arnold, G. Klingelschmitt, D. Masterman, P. Fontoura, S. Belachew, P. Chin, N. Mairon, H. Garren, L. Kappos, and OPERA I and OPERA II Clinical Investigators. 2017. Ocrelizumab versus interferon beta-

1a in relapsing multiple sclerosis. *New England Journal of Medicine* 376(3):221-234.

Hess, A., R. Axmann, J. Rech, S. Finzel, C. Heindl, S. Kreitz, M. Sergeeva, M. Saake, M. Garcia, G. Kollias, R. H. Straub, O. Sporns, A. Doerfler, K. Brune, and G. Schett. 2011. Blockade of TNF-alpha rapidly inhibits pain responses in the central nervous system. *Proceedings of the National Academy of Sciences* 108(9):3731-3736.

Hickman, S. E., N. D. Kingery, T. K. Ohsumi, M. L. Borowsky, L. C. Wang, T. K. Means, and J. El Khoury. 2013. The microglial sensome revealed by direct RNA sequencing. *Nature Neuroscience* 16(12):1896-1905.

Jay, T. R., C. M. Miller, P. J. Cheng, L. C. Graham, S. Bemiller, M. L. Broihier, G. Xu, D. Margevicius, J. C. Karlo, G. L. Sousa, A. C. Cotleur, O. Butovsky, L. Bekris, S. M. Staugaitis, J. B. Leverenz, S. W. Pimplikar, G. E. Landreth, G. R. Howell, R. M. Ransohoff, and B. T. Lamb. 2015. TREM2 deficiency eliminates TREM2+ inflammatory macrophages and ameliorates pathology in Alzheimer's disease mouse models. *Journal of Experimental Medicine* 212(3):287-295.

Khandaker, G. M., R. M. Pearson, S. Zammit, G. Lewis, and P. B. Jones. 2014. Association of serum interleukin 6 and C-reactive protein in childhood with depression and psychosis in young adult life: A population-based longitudinal study. *JAMA Psychiatry* 71(10):1121-1128.

Kirk, J., J. Plumb, M. Mirakhur, and S. McQuaid. 2003. Tight junctional abnormality in multiple sclerosis white matter affects all calibres of vessel and is associated with blood–brain barrier leakage and active demyelination. *The Journal of Pathology* 201(2):319-327.

Kreisl, W. C., C. H. Lyoo, M. McGwier, J. Snow, K. J. Jenko, N. Kimura, W. Corona, C. L. Morse, S. S. Zoghbi, V. W. Pike, F. J. McMahon, R. S. Turner, R. B. Innis, and Biomarkers Consortium PET Radioligand Project Team. 2013. In vivo radioligand binding to translocator protein correlates with severity of Alzheimer's disease. *Brain* 136(Pt 7):2228-2238.

Lee, J. W., H. Namkoong, H. K. Kim, S. Kim, D. W. Hwang, H. R. Na, S.-A. Ha, J.-R. Kim, and J. W. Kim. 2007. Fibrinogen gamma-A chain precursor in CSF: A candidate biomarker for Alzheimer's disease. *BMC Neurology* 7(14).

Li, R., A. Rezk, Y. Miyazaki, E. Hilgenberg, H. Touil, P. Shen, C. S. Moore, L. Michel, F. Althekair, S. Rajasekharan, J. L. Gommerman, A. Prat, S. Fillatreau, A. Bar-Or, and Canadian B Cells in MS Team. 2015. Proinflammatory GM-CSF-producing B cells in multiple sclerosis and B cell depletion therapy. *Science Translational Medicine* 7(310):310ra166.

Loane, D. J., and K. R. Byrnes. 2010. Role of microglia in neurotrauma. *Neurotherapeutics* 7(4):366-377.

Macosko, E. Z., A. Basu, R. Satija, J. Nemesh, K. Shekhar, M. Goldman, I. Tirosh, A. R. Bialas, N. Kamitaki, E. M. Martersteck, J. J. Trombetta, D. A. Weitz, J. R. Sanes, A. K. Shalek, A. Regev, and S. A. McCarroll. 2015. Highly parallel genome-wide expression profiling of individual cells using nanoliter droplets. *Cell* 161(5):1202-1214.

Magliozzi, R., O. W. Howell, C. Reeves, F. Roncaroli, R. Nicholas, B. Serafini, F. Aloisi, and R. Reynolds. 2010. A gradient of neuronal loss and meningeal inflammation in multiple sclerosis. *Annals of Neurology* 68(4):477-493.

Marik, C., P. A. Felts, J. Bauer, H. Lassmann, and K. J. Smith. 2007. Lesion genesis in a subset of patients with multiple sclerosis: a role for innate immunity? *Brain* 130(Pt 11):2800-2815.

McIntyre, R. S., D. S. Cha, J. M. Jerrell, W. Swardfager, R. D. Kim, L. G. Costa, A. Baskaran, J. K. Soczynska, H. O. Woldeyohannes, R. B. Mansur, E. Brietzke, A. M. Powell, A. Gallaugher, P. Kudlow, O. Kaidanovich-Beilin, and M. Alsuwaidan. 2014. Advancing biomarker research: Utilizing "big data" approaches for the characterization and prevention of bipolar disorder. *International Journal of Bipolar Disorders* 16(5):531-547.

Miller, A. H., and C. L. Raison. 2016. The role of inflammation in depression: From evolutionary imperative to modern treatment target. *Nature Reviews Immunology* 16(1):22-34.

Mouzon, B., H. Chaytow, G. Crynen, C. Bachmeier, J. Stewart, M. Mullan, W. Stewart, and F. Crawford. 2012. Repetitive mild traumatic brain injury in a mouse model produces learning and memory deficits accompanied by histological changes. *Journal of Neurotrauma* 29(18):2761-2773.

Mouzon, B. C., C. Bachmeier, A. Ferro, J. O. Ojo, G. Crynen, C. M. Acker, P. Davies, M. Mullan, W. Stewart, and F. Crawford. 2014. Chronic neuropathological and neurobehavioral changes in a repetitive mild traumatic brain injury model. *Annals of Neurology* 75(2):241-254.

Perrin, R. J., A. M. Fagan, and D. M. Holtzman. 2009. Multimodal techniques for diagnosis and prognosis of Alzheimer's disease. *Nature* 461(7266):916-922.

Raison, C. L., R. E. Rutherford, B. J. Woolwine, C. Shuo, P. Schettler, D. F. Drake, E. Haroon, and A. H. Miller. 2013. A randomized controlled trial of the tumor necrosis factor antagonist infliximab for treatment-resistant depression: The role of baseline inflammatory biomarkers. *JAMA Psychiatry* 70(1):31-41.

Ryu, J. K., and J. G. McLarnon. 2009. A leaky blood-brain barrier, fibrinogen infiltration and microglial reactivity in inflamed Alzheimer's disease brain. *Journal of Cellular and Molecular Medicine* 13(9A):2911-2925.

Ryu, J. K., M. A. Petersen, S. G. Murray, K. M. Baeten, A. Meyer-Franke, J. P. Chan, E. Vagena, C. Bedard, M. R. Machado, P. E. Rios Coronado, T. Prod'homme, I. F. Charo, H. Lassmann, J. L. Degen, S. S. Zamvil, and K. Akassoglou. 2015. Blood coagulation protein fibrinogen promotes autoimmunity and demyelination via chemokine release and antigen presentation. *Nature Communications* 6:8164.

Schachtrup, C., J. K. Ryu, M. J. Helmrick, E. Vagena, D. K. Galanakis, J. L. Degen, R. U. Margolis, and K. Akassoglou. 2010. Fibrinogen triggers astrocyte scar formation by promoting the availability of active TGF-beta after vascular damage. *Journal of Neuroscience* 30(17):5843-5854.

Sekar, A., A. R. Bialas, H. de Rivera, A. Davis, T. R. Hammond, N. Kamitaki, K. Tooley, J. Presumey, M. Baum, V. Van Doren, G. Genovese, S. A. Rose, R. E. Handsaker, Schizophrenia Working Group of the Psychiatric Genomics Consortium, M. J. Daly, M. C. Carroll, B. Stevens, and S. A. McCarroll. 2016. Schizophrenia risk from complex variation of complement component 4. *Nature* 530(7589):177-183.

Setiawan, E., A. A. Wilson, R. Mizrahi, P. M. Rusjan, L. Miler, G. Rajkowska, I. Suridjan, J. L. Kennedy, P. V. Rekkas, S. Houle, and J. H. Meyer. 2015. Role of translocator protein density, a marker of neuroinflammation, in the brain during major depressive episodes. *JAMA Psychiatry* 72(3):268-275.

Sieweke, M. H., and J. E. Allen. 2013. Beyond stem cells: Self-renewal of differentiated macrophages. *Science* 342(6161):1242974.

Streit, W. J., N. W. Sammons, A. J. Kuhns, and D. L. Sparks. 2004. Dystrophic microglia in the aging human brain. *Glia* 45(2):208-212.

Suarez-Calvet, M., M. A. Araque Caballero, G. Kleinberger, R. J. Bateman, A. M. Fagan, J. C. Morris, A. Danek, M. Ewers, C. Haass, and Dominantly Inherited Alzheimer Network. 2016. Early changes in CSF STREM2 in dominantly inherited Alzheimer's disease occur after amyloid deposition and neuronal injury. *Science Translational Medicine* 8(369):369ra178.

Tracey, K. J. 2002. The inflammatory reflex. *Nature* 420(6917):853-859.

Vos, C. M., J. J. Geurts, L. Montagne, E. S. van Haastert, L. Bo, P. van der Valk, F. Barkhof, and H. E. de Vries. 2005. Blood-brain barrier alterations in both focal and diffuse abnormalities on postmortem MRI in multiple sclerosis. *Neurobiology of Disease* 20(3):953-960.

Zhong, L., X. F. Chen, T. Wang, Z. Wang, C. Liao, Z. Wang, R. Huang, D. Wang, X. Li, L. Wu, L. Jia, H. Zheng, M. Painter, Y. Atagi, C. C. Liu, Y. W. Zhang, J. D. Fryer, H. Xu, and G. Bu. 2017. Soluble TREM2 induces inflammatory responses and enhances microglial survival. *Journal of Experimental Medicine* 214(3):597-607.

B

Workshop Agenda

BIOMARKERS OF NEUROINFLAMMATION: A WORKSHOP

March 20 and 21, 2017

National Academy of Sciences Building
2101 Constitution Avenue, NW | Washington, DC

Background: Innate and adaptive immunities have become very important areas of investigation for psychiatric disorders, neurological disorders, neurodevelopmental disorders, and neurodegeneration resulting from traumatic brain injury (TBI). For example, compelling genetic and other biological data are demonstrating critical roles of innate and adaptive immunity in Alzheimer's disease pathogenesis. Several conferences and meetings are being held in this hot area, but it is not clear how best to translate recent findings to therapeutics; developing biomarkers that can be validated and used in clinical development and regulatory decision making is a critical step in this process. Many efforts are already under way to identify biomarkers of neuroinflammation, including biomarkers in cerebrospinal fluid (CSF) and blood, as well as positron emission tomography imaging agents for targets such as translocator protein. Given the intense activity in academic research and private-sector settings and across many nervous system disorders, there is an opportunity to take stock of current knowledge, provide a venue for coordination, and identify potential opportunities to advance work in this domain. This public workshop will bring together key stakeholders from government, academia, industry, and disease-focused organizations to explore and advance efforts to identify biomarkers of neuroinflammation that can be validated and used in clinical development and regulatory decision making.

Workshop Objectives:

- Provide an overview of current knowledge on the role of neuroinflammation in nervous system disorders—including psychiatric and neurological disorders, neurodevelopmental disorders, and neurodegeneration resulting from TBI—discuss the various definitions of neuroinflammation in use across the field, and the contribution of the peripheral and central nervous system (CNS) innate immune systems to normal brain function and disease pathophysiology.
- Explore the state of the science of neuroinflammation biomarkers and research needed to enable the use of these biomarkers at the individual level. Do any biomarkers undergoing development/validation implicate glia, neurons, immune cells, and/or endothelial cells? Should these be deployed singly or in combination, and where are the gaps in current approaches?
- Facilitate coordination among consortia and companies that are developing biomarkers of neuroinflammation. How might a study be designed to establish the disease relevance or drug-development utility of a neuroinflammation biomarker? Are such studies under way, and if not, why not? If not, what more do we need to facilitate these, and are there opportunities for "add-on" studies to current clinical trials?
- Highlight approaches, tools, and lessons learned that may apply across disorders and opportunities to advance the development of these biomarkers.

DAY 1: March 20, 2017, Room 120

1:00 p.m.   **Welcome and Overview of Workshop**
RITA BALICE-GORDON, Sanofi (*Co-Chair*)
LINDA BRADY, National Institute of Mental Health (*Co-Chair*)

SESSION 1: STATE OF THE SCIENCE OF NEUROINFLAMMATION IN CNS DISORDERS

Session Objectives:
- Provide brief background information on inflammatory processes and the role of neuroinflammation in adaptive repair and protection as well as pathophysiology of the brain.
- Survey current knowledge on the role of neuroinflammation in nervous system disorders—including psychiatric and neurological disorders, and neurodegeneration resulting from TBI—and common pathways for neuroinflammation across different disorders.
- Discuss desirable biomarker characteristics for quantitatively tracking neuroinflammation in disease progression and therapeutic interventions in different CNS disorders.

1:15 p.m.	**Session Overview and Introduction** BRIAN CAMPBELL, MindImmune Therapeutics, Inc., and The University of Rhode Island (*Moderator*)
1:35 p.m.	**The Acute-to-Chronic Neuroinflammation Continuum** FIONA CRAWFORD, Roskamp Institute AMIT BAR-OR, University of Pennsylvania GARY LANDRETH, Case Western Reserve University
2:50 p.m.	**Break**
3:05 p.m.	**The Acute-to-Chronic Neuroinflammation Continuum (continued)** BETH STEVENS, Boston Children's Hospital RICHARD DANEMAN, University of California, San Diego
3:55 p.m.	**Discussion**
5:00 p.m.	**Adjourn Day 1**

DAY 2: March 21, 2017, Room 125

8:30 a.m.	**Welcome and Review of Day 1** RITA BALICE-GORDON, Sanofi (*Co-Chair*) LINDA BRADY, National Institute of Mental Health (*Co-Chair*)
8:40 a.m.	**Keynote Presentation** EDWARD BULLMORE, University of Cambridge and GlaxoSmithKline
9:10 a.m.	**Discussion** PATRICIO O'DONNELL, Pfizer Neuroscience Research Unit (*Moderator*)
9:30 a.m.	**Break**

SESSION 2: NEUROIMAGING BIOMARKERS—CURRENT INITIATIVES AND OPPORTUNITIES

Session Objectives:
- Discuss current consortia, academic, and private-sector efforts to identify and validate imaging biomarkers of neuroinflammation and share methodological approaches and lessons learned.
- Describe the use of neuroimaging biomarkers to identify changes in structure or tissue properties with respect to inflammation.
- Address key issues relevant across CNS disorders, such as the following:
    - How well do neuroimaging methods differentiate between adaptive and pathological neuroinflammatory processes?
    - Are current imaging agents useful in identifying specific patient populations?
    - What is the potential clinical utility of imaging agents and can they detect immediate and longer-term changes following therapeutic interventions?
- Describe the limitations of current imaging biomarkers of neuroinflammation and identify research and other potential next steps that would move the field forward.

APPENDIX B 67

9:45 a.m.   **Session Overview**
            ANNA KATRIN SZARDENINGS, Johnson & Johnson (*Moderator*)

9:55 a.m.   **Presentations**
            ANNA KATRIN SZARDENINGS, Johnson & Johnson
            ROBERT INNIS, National Institute of Mental Health
            MARTINA ABSINTA, National Institute of Neurological Disorders and Stroke
            KATERINA AKASSOGLOU, Gladstone Institute of Neurological Disease

11:10 a.m. **Discussion**

11:35 a.m. **Lunch**

SESSION 3: CSF AND OTHER FLUID BIOMARKERS—CURRENT INITIATIVES AND OPPORTUNITIES

Session Objectives:
- Discuss current consortia, academic, and private-sector efforts to identify and validate CSF and other fluid biomarkers of neuroinflammation and share methodological approaches and lessons learned.
- Address key issues relevant across CNS disorders, such as the following:
  o How well can CSF and other fluid biomarker detection methods differentiate between adaptive and pathological neuroinflammatory processes?
  o Are fluid biomarkers useful in identifying specific patient populations?
  o What is the potential clinical utility of fluid biomarkers and can they detect immediate and longer-term changes following therapeutic interventions?
  o How reliable are peripheral biomarkers as indicators of neuroinflammation?

- Describe the limitations of current fluid biomarkers of neuroinflammation and identify research and other potential next steps that would move the field forward.
- Explore the relationship between fluid and imaging biomarkers.

12:35 p.m. **Session Overview**
ELIEZER MASLIAH, National Institute on Aging (*Moderator*)

12:45 p.m. **Presentations**
BRIAN CAMPBELL, MindImmune Therapeutics, Inc., and The University of Rhode Island
RICHARD PERRIN, Washington University in St. Louis
STEVEN MCCARROLL, Harvard Medical School

1:45 p.m. **Discussion**

2:10 p.m. **Break**

SESSION 4: MOVING FORWARD

Session Objectives:
- Highlight key themes from the workshop.
- Discuss approaches, tools, and lessons learned that may apply across disorders and opportunities to advance the development of these biomarkers.
- Identify specific barriers and opportunities for increased coordinating among ongoing efforts in academia, the private sector, and consortia.
- Brainstorm potential collaborative projects that could be submitted through the Biomarkers Consortium or other current or planned mechanisms.
- Consider potential regulatory issues for biomarkers of neuroinflammation as research, development, and validation move forward.

2:25 p.m.	**Session Overview**
	    LINDA BRADY, National Institute of Mental Health
	    RITA BALICE-GORDON, Sanofi

2:35 p.m.	**Panel Remarks**
	    EDWARD BULLMORE, University of Cambridge and GlaxoSmithKline
	    GARY LANDRETH, Case Western Reserve University
	    RICHARD PERRIN, Washington University in St. Louis
	    AMIT BAR-OR, University of Pennsylvania
	    ANNA KATRIN SZARDENINGS, Johnson & Johnson
	    ANDREW MILLER, Emory University
	    TAREK SAMAD, Pfizer Inc.

3:45 p.m.	**Discussion**
4:30 p.m.	**Adjourn Workshop**

C
Registered Attendees

Martina Absinta
National Institute of Neurological Disorders and Stroke

Neeraj Agarwal
National Eye Institute

Katerina Akassoglou
Gladstone Institute of Neurological Disease

Shelli Avenevoli
National Institute of Mental Health

Lisa Bain
Lisa Bain, LLC

Rita Balice-Gordon
Sanofi

Amit Bar-Or
University of Pennsylvania

Luca Bartolini
Children's National Health System

Lizbet Boroughs
Association of American Universities

Linda Brady
National Institute of Mental Health

Andrew Breeden
National Institutes of Health

Emery Brown
Massachusetts Institute of Technology

Janet Brownlees
MRC Technology

Edward Bullmore
University of Cambridge
GlaxoSmithKline

Gregory Busse
Takeda Pharmaceuticals

Joseph Buxbaum
Icahn School of Medicine at Mount Sinai

Sarah Caddick
The Gatsby Charitable Foundation

Brian Campbell
MindImmune Therapeutics, Inc.
The University of Rhode Island

Rosa Canet-Aviles
Foundation of the National Institutes of Health

Kevin Champaigne
Clemson University

Sanjay Chandriani
BioMarin

Wen Chen
National Center for Complementary and Integrative Health

E. Antonio Chiocca
Brigham and Women's Hospital

Angela Christian
Independent Writer/Editor

Roderick Corriveau
National Institute of Neurological Disorders and Stroke

Fiona Crawford
Roskamp Institute

Changhai Cui
National Institute on Alcohol Abuse and Alcoholism

Richard Daneman
University of California, San Diego

Bernard Dardzinski
Uniformed Services University of the Health Sciences

Thomas DeGraba
National Intrepid Center of Excellence

Joan Demetriades
One Mind

Nancy Desmond
National Institute of Mental Health

Ramon Diaz-Arrastia
University of Pennsylvania

Amanda DiBattista
National Institute on Aging

APPENDIX C 73

Wayne Drevets
Janssen Research & Development, LLC

Emmeline Edwards
National Center for Complementary and Integrative Health

Scott Fogerty
Thermo Fisher Scientific/ Diagnostic Partnering

Allyson Gage
Cohen Veterans Bioscience

Yurong Gao
Food and Drug Administration

Aarti Gautam
U.S. Army Medical Research and Materiel Command

Joshua Gordon
National Institute of Mental Health

Christopher Gorini
Food and Drug Administration

Paula Grammas
The University of Rhode Island

Henry Greely
Stanford University

Michelle Guignet
University of California, Davis

Anthony Hardie
Veterans for Common Sense

Dean Hartley
Alzheimer's Association

Brian Harvey
Brian E. Harvey, LLC

Miles Herkenham
National Institute of Mental Health

Mi Hillefors
National Institute of Mental Health

Richard Hodes
National Institutes of Health

Stuart Hoffman
Department of Veterans Affairs

John Hsiao
National Institute on Aging

Amanda Hunt
Department of Veterans Affairs

Steven Hyman
Stanley Center for Psychiatric Research

Robert Innis
National Institute of Mental Health

Frances Jensen
University of Pennsylvania Perelman School of Medicine

Sophia Jeon
Kelly Government Solutions/ National Institute of Neurological Disorders and Stroke

Marti Jett
U.S. Army Medical Research and Materiel Command

Jeymohan Joseph
National Institute of Mental Health

David Kaplan
CellPrint Biotechnology

Nicholas Kaye
CellPrint Biotechnology

Kimbra Kenney
National Intrepid Center of Excellence

Hartmuth Kolb
Janssen R&D San Diego

Walter Koroshetz
National Institute of Neurological Disorders and Stroke

Lina Kubli
Department of Veterans Affairs

David Kulick
Quanterix

Story Landis
National Institute of Neurological Disorders and Stroke

Gary Landreth
Indiana University School of Medicine

Alan Leshner
American Association for the Advancement of Science

Marilyn Lightfoote
Food and Drug Administration

Yuan Luo
National Institute on Aging

Mack Mackiewicz
National Institute on Aging

Andrea Horvath Marques
National Institute of Mental Health

Zane Martin
National Institutes of Health

Terina Martinez
The Michael J. Fox
  Foundation for Parkinson's
  Research

Eliezer Masliah
National Institute on Aging

Steven McCarroll
Harvard Medical School

Kristina McLinden
National Institute on Aging

Enrique Michelotti
National Institute of Mental
  Health

Andrew Miller
Emory University

Bradley Miller
Eli Lilly and Company

Marilyn Miller
National Institutes of Health

David Millis
Food and Drug
  Administration

Christian Mirescu
Merck Research Labs

Thomas Möller
AbbVie Foundational
  Neuroscience Center

Richard Nakamura
Center for Scientific Review,
  National Institutes of Health

Robert Nelson
MindImmune, Inc.

Montra Denise Nichols
U.S. Air Force (Ret.)

Antonio Noronha
National Institute on Alcohol
  Abuse and Alcoholism

Patricio O'Donnell
Pfizer Inc.

Lisa Opanashuk
National Institute on Aging

Carlos Peña
Food and Drug
  Administration

Richard Perrin
Washington University in
  St. Louis

Creighton Phelps
National Institute on Aging
  (Ret.)

William Potter
National Institute of Mental
  Health

Allison Provost
Cohen Veterans Bioscience

Deepa Rao
Food and Drug
　Administration

Vasudev Rao
National Institute of Mental
　Health

William Renehan
The University of Rhode
　Island

John Reppa
Neurotechnology Industry
　Organization

Lucille Roberts
National Institute on Aging

Tarek Samad
Pfizer Inc.

Kathryn Sanchez
Georgetown University

Joshua Sanes
Harvard University

Joseph Santoro
The Atlantic

Samantha Scott
National Institutes of Health

Christian Shenoua
Food and Drug
　Administration

David Shurtleff
National Center for
　Complementary and
　Integrative Health

Marni Silverman
Uniformed Services
　University of the Health
　Sciences

Kay Smith
Medical/Scientific Consultant

Martha Somerman
National Institute of Dental
　and Craniofacial Research

Beth Stevens
Harvard Medical School

Margaret Sutherland
National Institute of
　Neurological Disorders and
　Stroke

Anna-Katrin Szardenings
Janssen Research &
　Development

Amir Tamiz
National Institute of
　Neurological Disorders and
　Stroke

Nadine Tatton
Association for
　Frontotemporal
　Degeneration

Jean Tiong-Koehler
National Institute on Aging

Hao Wang
Takeda Pharmaceuticals

Hong Wang
Eli Lilly and Company

Alan Willard
National Institute of Neurological Disorders and Stroke

Lois Winsky
National Institute of Mental Health

Bradley C. Wise
National Institute on Aging